Diana K. Harris
Michael L. Benson

Maltreatment of Patients in Nursing Homes
There Is No Safe Place

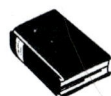

*Pre-publication
REVIEWS,
COMMENTARIES,
EVALUATIONS . . .*

"**A**n insightful view of what is really happening in nursing home facilities. The authors clearly describe the factors that conspire to make theft a common form of elder abuse. The residents' complaints are often ignored by staff and administrators and instead are attributed to symptoms of dementia. The result is a secondary form of abuse, as residents feel confused and even more vulnerable.

The suggestions for staff training and empowerment are superb and right on the mark! This book should be required reading for facility administrators, staff development personnel, and gerontology training programs."

Stacey Wood, PhD
*Assistant Professor of Psychology,
Scripps College*

"**T**his book is both chilling and fascinating. It substantiates what many of us have long suspected: that the safety of our loved ones, and perhaps eventually ourselves, cannot be guaranteed by placement in a nursing home. As the authors clearly demonstrate, sometimes nursing homes provide the ideal setting for the commission of every imaginable variety of crime from intentional neglect to murder. Criminal motives, helpless victims, and moments of opportunity often have tragic results.

Although this book paints a dark picture of the harm that may occur in nursing homes, it also provides pragmatic recommendations for screening out potential abusers and increasing the support and recognition for caring, hardworking staff devoted to improving the quality of life for all residents. This book is a must-read for anyone who has a loved one either in, or anticipating, nursing home placement, and for all of us who are growing older and may someday need care ourselves."

Joanne M. Otto, MSW
*Executive Director, National Adult
Protective Services Association*

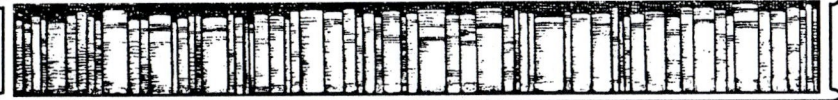

More pre-publication
REVIEWS, COMMENTARIES, EVALUATIONS . . .

"*Maltreatment of Patients in Nursing Homes* is an excellent read that will be of interest to many different groups. Addressing the kinds of offenses perpetrated against nursing home residents will make this book appealing to families of nursing home residents as well as the residents themselves. Describing the reasons these offenses occur will make the work useful to nursing home workers (staff and administrators alike). By tying in criminological theories, the book will be useful for criminologists wanting to research issues about victims or teach about these topics in their courses. Students in these courses will have their minds opened to a topic that likely has not been on their radar. Gerontologists and other social scientists will find value in the broad brush the authors paint with in describing these issues. Finally, policymakers will find value in the implications and recommendations that arise out of this work. Anyone interested in crime and victimization should read this book."

Brian K. Payne, PhD
Chair and Professor,
Sociology and Criminal Justice;
Director, Center for Family
Violence Education and Research,
Old Dominion University

The Haworth Pastoral Press®
An Imprint of The Haworth Press, Inc.
New York • London • Oxford

Maltreatment of Patients in Nursing Homes
There Is No Safe Place

THE HAWORTH PASTORAL PRESS®
Religion and Mental Health
Harold G. Koenig, MD
Senior Editor

Maltreatment of Patients in Nursing Homes
There Is No Safe Place

Diana K. Harris
Michael L. Benson

The Haworth Pastoral Press®
An Imprint of The Haworth Press, Inc.
New York • London • Oxford

For more information on this book or to order, visit
http://www.haworthpress.com/store/product.asp?sku=5461

or call 1-800-HAWORTH (800-429-6784) in the United States and Canada
or (607) 722-5857 outside the United States and Canada

or contact orders@HaworthPress.com

Published by

The Haworth Pastoral Press®, an imprint of The Haworth Press, Inc., 10 Alice Street, Binghamton, NY 13904-1580.

PUBLISHER'S NOTE
Identities and circumstances of individuals discussed in this book have been changed to protect confidentiality.

Nursing home photos by Nick Myers.

Cover design by Kerry E. Mack.

Library of Congress Cataloging-in-Publication Data

Harris, Diana K.
  Maltreatment of patients in nursing homes : there is no safe place / Diana K. Harris, Michael L. Benson.
      p. cm.
Includes bibliographical references and index.
    ISBN-13: 978-0-7890-2325-4 (hc. : alk. paper)
    ISBN-10: 0-7890-2325-3 (hc. : alk. paper)
    ISBN-13: 978-0-7890-2326-1 (pbk. : alk. paper)
    ISBN-10: 0-7890-2326-1 (pbk. : alk. paper)
    1. Nursing home patients—Abuse of—United States. 2. Nursing homes—Corrupt practices—United States. 3. Tort liability of nursing homes—United States. 4. Older people—Nursing home care—United States. 5. Older people—Abuse of—United States—Prevention. 6. Theft—United States. I. Benson, Michael L. II. Title.
    [DNLM: 1. Homes for the Aged—organization & administration—United States. 2. Nursing Homes—organization & administration—United States. 3. Elder Abuse—prevention & control—United States. 4. Nurses' Aides—organization & Administration—United States. 5. Patient Rights—legislation & jurisprudence—Aged—United States. 6. Theft—legislation & jurisprudence—United States.]

RA997.H357 2005
362.16—dc22

                                                                        2005003564

CONTENTS

PART IV: FRAUD, REFORM, AND RECOMMENDATIONS

ABOUT THE AUTHORS

Diana K. Harris, MA, co-directed the first national study on the theft of possessions belonging to nursing home patients. She is a past recipient of the National Alumni Public Service Award for her work with the elderly and has been honored by the National University Continuing Education Association for her independent study courses "Working with the Elderly" and "Problems of Aging and Retirement." Ms. Harris founded the Cole Council on Aging at the University of Tennessee in 1979, serving as its chairperson until 1991.

Ms. Harris is the Author of *The Sociology of Aging, The Elderly in American Society, The Sociology of Aging: An Annotated Bibliography and Sourcebook,* and the *Dictionary of Gerontology.* She also served from 1989-2000 as Series Editor for Garland Publishing, Inc., for their Issues in Aging series and was an Associate Editor for the *Encyclopedia of Ageism* (Haworth).

Michael L. Benson, PhD, is Professor of Criminal Justice at the University of Cincinnati in Ohio. He has been published extensively in leading academic journals on the issues of white-collar crime, domestic violence, and elder abuse. Dr. Benson received the Outstanding Scholar Award from the Crime and Juvenile Delinquency Division of the Society for the Study of Social Problems for his book *Combating Corporate Crime.*

Preface

This book is unique in two ways. One is that it contains the first and only nationwide study of theft from patients in nursing homes. With the exception of the work done by the authors, systematic research dealing with nursing home theft has been nonexistent. The second way this book is unique is that, to date, most books about elder abuse have dealt primarily with abuse in domestic settings. This is one of the first books to deal exclusively with the abuse of patients in nursing homes.

The book has been divided into four parts. Part I provides information about nursing homes and nursing aides, and discusses some of the theories regarding abuse. Part II deals with the thieves in nursing homes and the victims' families, and concludes with strategies to prevent and decrease theft. Part III focuses on physical and psychological abuse and suggests some ways to reduce these practices. Finally, Part IV discusses additional ways in which nursing home patients are maltreated, including financial abuse and violation of rights.

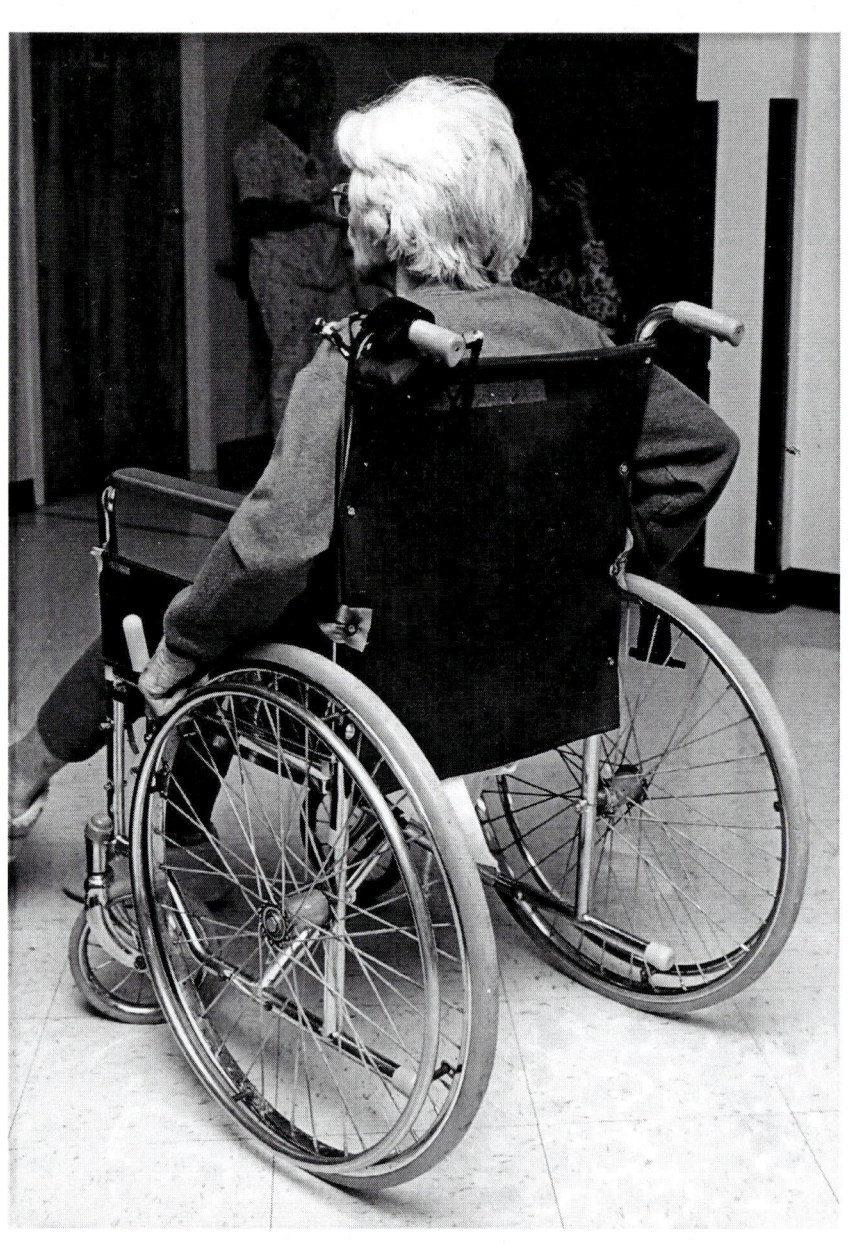

PART I:
NURSING HOMES
AND THEORIES OF ABUSE

Chapter 1

The Nature of Nursing Homes

If you are over the age of fifty, the chances are pretty good that you know someone who is or soon will be in a **nursing home**. It could be a parent or grandparent, an aunt or uncle, a spouse, or even yourself.

In the past few decades, the nursing home has become for many people a much feared but seemingly unavoidable part of aging and growing old. The fear, anxiety, and trepidation that most of us feel at the prospect of sending a loved one (or going ourselves) to a nursing home is, of course, understandable. Being admitted to a nursing home signifies in a depressingly formal and institutional way that a person is entering the final stages of life. It is a significant transition in the life course. It means giving up your home, your surroundings, and a lifetime's accumulation of possessions that make you feel connected, secure, and comfortable.

Despite the fear and anxiety that they provoke in many people, nursing homes nevertheless now play a vital role in our nation's health care system. As we will discuss, in the not-too-distant past when a parent or spouse became unable to take care of themselves, someone in their immediate family would care for them. Few facilities specifically designed for long-term care of the aged existed. But in today's geographically mobile world, children often live far away from their parents. Even if they live nearby, many families are simply unable to care for an aging parent, perhaps because both the husband and the wife work. Thus, when parents become ill or senile or simply unable to care for themselves, it can be an overwhelming burden on their children, who have their own lives to lead.

Nursing homes can be a godsend to families unable to meet the health care needs of their elderly members. They can provide round-the-clock medical care, which may extend a person's life years beyond what would be possible if he or she stayed in the community.

Hence, when the ability to function independently in the community is lost, many families have no other option but to put their loved one and their trust in a nursing home.

The decision to entrust the care of a loved one to the staff and management of a nursing home usually is well intentioned. Certainly, most facilities try to do a good job. Certainly, a large majority of the people who work in nursing homes are dedicated and caring individuals who do the best they can to maintain and improve the quality of life of their charges. But not *every* nursing home is perfect and not *every* employee keeps the commitment to serve their patients' needs. Sadly, some individuals violate both their duty to their patients and the trust that families have placed in them. These individuals abuse and take advantage of their patients. There is, then, a dark side to nursing homes, and this book is about that dark side.

We have decided to write about the dark side of nursing homes for several reasons. Given the large number of individuals who spend at least some time in a nursing home, the problem of **abuse** in nursing homes potentially affects many people. The people affected by abuse in nursing homes are among the most vulnerable victims in society. They are old, weak, and often cognitively impaired. They are unable to stand up for themselves. Despite the potential importance of abuse in nursing homes as a social problem, surprisingly little research on this topic exists. Hence, another reason for writing this book is to bring together what is known about nursing home abuse and offer it to the general population. Although it is a difficult and depressing topic to investigate, some researchers have made efforts to chart its extent and variety. We aim to summarize what is currently known and to point out what questions still need answers. We also hope that by shedding light on the issue of abuse in nursing homes we can spur efforts by lawmakers and by the industry to ameliorate the problem. Finally, we hope this book will help the families of nursing home patients and ultimately the patients themselves by educating them about an issue that is often ignored and trivialized.

MYTHS AND FACTS ABOUT NURSING HOMES

The following are some widely held views and commonsense notions about nursing homes and their patients and personnel. As you read through these statements, you might want to write down whether you think they are true or false.

Most persons age sixty-five and over live in nursing homes because they are unable to care for themselves.

False. Although it sounds reasonable, this actually is a misconception. The truth is that a majority of older persons live in the community. It is estimated that just under 6 percent, 1.5 million, of the older population live in a nursing home on any given day (Mitty, 2001). However, 20 percent of all males and 34 percent of all females can expect to experience at least one nursing home stay in their lifetime (American Health Care Association, 2001).

The cost of living in a nursing home is covered by Medicare.

False. Contrary to popular belief, **Medicare** contributes little— only about 9 percent—to nursing home care. Medicare, a national health insurance program for people age sixty-five and over, will pay for the first twenty days of approved skilled care in a nursing home *after hospitalization.* It then pays a portion of the cost for days 21 to 100. However, **Medicaid** coverage is available to eligible low-income persons and to nursing home patients who have exhausted their own resources paying for nursing home care. Medicaid, a health insurance program jointly funded by the federal and state governments, pays for the care provided to about two-thirds of nursing home patients nationwide.

Long-term care and nursing home care are one and the same.

False. **Long-term care** is assistance given over a period of time to those who have difficulty in functioning because of a chronic disability. Such care is mostly given by family members and friends, while nursing home care refers to a residential facility that routinely provides nursing-care services.

Most people in the nursing home population are women.

True. Women make up more than two-thirds of nursing home patients. The typical nursing home patient is white, female, a Medicaid beneficiary, and seventy-five years of age or older.

As in hospitals, highly trained nurses provide most of the care in nursing homes.

False. Nursing home aides (also called nurse assistants, or certified nursing aides) are responsible for 80 to 90 percent of patient care in nursing homes. Although they are supervised by nurses, most of the work with patients in nursing homes is done by aides who have relatively little training and who are ill-prepared for the stresses of working with nursing home patients.

Most nursing homes are nonprofit organizations.

False. About 67 percent are for profit, 26 percent are nonprofit, and 7 percent are government owned and operated. It is estimated that the industry generates close to $80 billion in revenues each year.

Many of the people in nursing homes suffer from dementia.

True. Close to half of all nursing home patients suffer from some form of cognitive impairment. **Dementia** refers to a decline in mental functioning, which includes impairment of memory, orientation, and judgment.

Most long-term care is provided by nursing homes.

False. Even though the number of nursing homes and the size of the nursing home population are growing, about 80 percent of long-term care is provided by family, friends, and volunteers.

The older you become, the more likely you are to live in a nursing home.

True. Individuals eighty-five and older constitute the largest age group in nursing homes. They make up nearly half of the nursing home population.

No one looks out for the interests of nursing home patients, except their families.

False. All states have at least one full-time **ombudsperson**. An ombudsperson is an advocate who is responsible for investigating and resolving complaints on behalf of patients in nursing homes and other long-term care facilities. In addition, thousands of trained volunteer ombudspersons regularly visit long-term care facilities to monitor conditions and care.

Most nursing home patients are single or never married.

False. More than 60 percent are widowed.

No uniform data on the prevalence of abuse in nursing homes exist.

True. However, abuses have been documented in government reports, ethnographic studies, and ombudsman projects. The findings suggest that abuse of nursing home patients may be even more extensive than is generally thought.

The workforce of persons employed in nursing homes consists mainly of females.

True. In 1998, according to the Bureau of Labor Statistics, 85 percent of the workforce was female. (Twenty-four percent of the entire workforce were black and 7.4 percent were Hispanic.)

Most nursing aides are poorly paid.

True. The work of these minimum-wage workers has been described as "low tech and high touch." They also comprise the largest number of positions in all nursing homes.

The state with the largest number of nursing homes is Florida.

False. California has the largest number of nursing homes (1,378) followed by Texas (1,251), while Florida has 734 facilities. The total number of nursing homes in the United States is about 17,000.

The cost of nursing home care is more expensive than most people realize.

True. Nationally, the average cost per month is about $4,600.

Abuse of patients in nursing homes often goes unreported.

True. Often, patients and family members are reluctant to complain; many fear that complaints will result in retaliation by the staff.

This book deals exclusively with nursing homes, the most common type of residential care facility. Other types include board-and-care homes, group homes, homes for the aged, adult foster care homes, **assisted living facilities,** and adult congregate living. A nursing home may be defined as a facility with three or more beds that is licensed by the state as a nursing home and is usually certified for federal reimbursement as a Medicaid and/or skilled Medicare nursing facility.

HOW NURSING HOMES GOT STARTED

Prior to 1935, few facilities for the aged existed. The majority of the aged who could not provide for themselves and had no family to help them generally lived in public facilities such as homes for the aged, mental institutions, and **almshouses,** which were popularly referred to as "poor farms," "county homes," or "poor houses." In 1871 Will Carleton wrote about the plight of a homeless aged woman without means. The famous ballad began, "Over the hill to the poor house I'm trudgin' my weary way . . ." The first three words, "over the hill," are commonly used today to denote someone who is superannuated.

Besides almshouses, other alternatives that preceded the establishment of nursing homes were private homes for the aged run by charitable organizations and private proprietary boarding homes for those able to pay. As the need for nursing care arose among the residents of the homes for the aged and boarding homes, many of these facilities added nursing staff and gradually evolved into nursing homes or personal care homes with infirmaries. The real boost to these two settings, however, came with the passage of the Social Security Act of 1935 (Dunlop, 1979).

The Social Security Act, with its Old Age Assistance (OAA) provision, greatly increased the number of persons who could afford to move to private facilities run for profit. However, at that time, recipients of OAA were considered ineligible to collect monthly benefits if they were inmates of a public facility. The denying of OAA payments to older people who lived in public institutions forced many chronically ill elderly to move into boarding homes and private homes that capitalized on the newly moneyed aged population, who could now pay with OAA funds. In time, these places began to call themselves "nursing homes." Unintentionally, then, Social Security was responsible for the growth of the nursing home industry.

The passage of the Medicare/Medicaid Bill in 1965 gave the nursing home industry another big boost in growth because of the large infusion of public funds into private facilities, which made public homes virtually obsolete. As noted earlier, Medicaid pays the cost of nursing home care for low-income persons or for those who have used up their finances paying nursing home costs, while Medicare helps pay nursing home costs up to 100 days after hospitalization. For a nursing home to be certified to receive Medicare and Medicaid payments, it must comply with federal regulations concerning the patients' quality of life and care. As a result, nursing homes are periodically inspected to determine if they meet federal certification and state licensing regulations. This modification in the health care financing system, together with the increasing demand for beds as the number of elderly persons has increased, accounts for most of the current growth in the nursing home population.

Although the number of elderly persons in nursing homes has continued to increase, the rate of increase has been slower in recent years. This decline may be due in part to the greater use of home-based care and assisted living facilities. Currently, about 1.7 million nursing home patients exist in the United States. It is projected that by 2050 the number is expected to rise to 6.6 million, as the baby boomers become elderly and life expectancy continues to increase (American Health Care Association, 2001). Table 1.1 provides some information on the demographic characteristics of the nursing home population.

What Do You Call Persons Living in Nursing Homes?

For those who live in nursing homes the nomenclature problem is often finessed by the term *resident*. This is hardly a solution, however; people who reside in nursing homes and other residential settings are *patients* with reference to their health care providers but can be thought of as residents or tenants in relation to those who supply their housing. But since people in nursing homes are treated like patients, "patients" is the more preferable term to use. (Kane et al., 1998, p. 5)

NURSING HOMES AS BUREAUCRACIES

Large, impersonal formal organizations are called **bureaucracies** and they dominant our society today. Bureaucracies have a chain of command or hierarchy of authority that operates under definite rules and procedures. According to the famous German sociologist Max Weber (1922), bureaucracies typically have a clear-cut division of labor and members, who have specialized jobs to do, take orders from the persons immediately above them in the hierarchy. Examples of bureaucracies include factories, business corporations, and universities. Even though nursing homes are small organizations, they manifest many of the properties of bureaucratic structures. In theory, they are rationally designed for the greatest efficiency and the achievement of specific objectives. In a typical nursing home, the chain of command or hierarchy consists of a nursing home administrator and a

TABLE 1.1. Nursing Home Patients by Selected Demographic Characteristics, 1999

Characteristic	Percent
Age	
Under 65	9.8
65 and over	90.3
65-74	12.0
75-84	31.8
85 and over	46.5
Sex	
Female	71.9
Male	28.1
Race	
White	85.7
Black	11.0
Marital Status	
Married	17.6
Widowed	57.4
Divorced or separated	8.4
Single or never married	15.0

Source: Jones (2000).

medical director at the top level. The administrator is responsible for directing and coordinating all activities of the home in order to carry out its objectives in providing patient care. The medical director plans and coordinates patient care in establishing standards of medical service. At the next highest level in the caregiving department is the director of nurses, who is responsible for the administration of nursing services, followed by an assistant director of nurses and nursing supervisors who coordinate the activities of personnel assigned to a specific shift. Other positions include staff nurses, charge nurses, and practical nurses. At the bottom of the hierarchy are **nursing aides**. The larger a formal organization becomes, the more it needs bureaucratic practices to coordinate its members' activities.

A bureaucracy relies on highly rationalized procedures to achieve specific objectives. For example, the major objectives in a nursing home are to ensure proper care of the patients and help prevent abuse and **neglect**. All the employees have specialized jobs to do and they concentrate on specific tasks. For example, Gubrium (1975) refers to the nursing aides' normal work routine as "bed-and-body work." He notes that the aides believe that once beds have been made and the highly visible bodily needs of the patients have been attended to, the staff has done its day's work. Nursing aides must adhere to rigid schedules in order to finish these tasks in the allotted time. Those who fall behind because they take the time to respond to patients' special needs are often chastised. One nursing aide explains why it is important to stop and talk to the patients even though aides are always overburdened and in a hurry, trying to get their chores done:

> There are people that don't have families or don't get visitors most of the time, so they rather enjoy you taking the time to talk to them or be with them to listen to them. Some people feel like talking, but when there is nobody to listen to them they feel very bad, so sometimes I sit with them, I talk to them. (O'Brien, 1989, p. 111)

Adhering to rigid schedules not only puts the staff under pressure, but also restricts the patients' freedom—even to the point of when they can go to the bathroom, if help is needed. In nursing homes, other people control the fundamental features of one's daily lifestyle and the **autonomy** of a patient is highly restricted. A formal routine is often prescribed for getting up (morning starts extremely early, sometimes at 5:30 a.m.), as well as going to bed and eating meals. Staff members tend to focus on routine and efficiency. They must care for large numbers of frail, dependent people, sometimes in an "assembly-line" manner. Respect for the rights of individual patients sometimes gets lost in the drive to operate efficiently as a business (Burger et al., 2000).

By now you might be wondering why bureaucracy is so necessary. The answer is simple: In an organization such as a nursing home, without bureaucracy, chaos would result. The bureaucratic form of organization thrives because it is the best means ever devised for a business to function effectively and efficiently. Foner (1994) notes that "Nursing home workers cannot simply 'do their own thing'. . . while some undoubtedly would do a good job without formal rules and clearly-defined duties many others would not" (p. 55).

Nursing Homes and Bureaucracy

Families and residents experience bureaucracy in a variety of ways including: the routinized, sometimes "assembly-line" nature of care routines; the highly regulated hierarchy of information exchange and authority within the staff; and the prominence of rules and procedures over negotiated relationships as guides for behavior. (Brannon, 1992)

NURSING HOMES AS TOTAL INSTITUTIONS

Nursing homes are not only bureaucratic entities but also are considered to be **"total institutions."** According to Erving Goffman (1961), such institutions are places of residence where a large number of like-situated individuals are cut off from the wider society for an appreciable length of time. The "inmates" lead enclosed, formally administered lives in that all aspects and activities of daily life are tightly scheduled and regulated by a hierarchy of custodians. As a result, all activities are conducted in the same place and the "inmates" are usually treated in groups and required to do the same thing together.

Total institutions are "total" because they completely control the life's of their residents. This is achieved by ritualized processes of initiation (nursing home admission) and degradation (loss of privacy, submission to rules). Thus, residents' identities are first stripped away and then reconstituted within the institutional system; a person becomes a resident, who is defined by his or her age along with specific medical diagnoses. By complying with the rules, residents can gain privileges; non-compliance leads to negative outcomes. Total institutions render their inhabitants quite vulnerable to any negative behaviors on the part of

> the institutional personnel. (Pasupathi and Lockenhoff, 2002 p. 211)

Entry into a total institution not only requires a restructuring of one's way of life, loss of freedom and independence, and an acquisition of institutional values, but it is also a process of transition in which people give up their former roles. For example, nursing home patients are no longer able to perform the roles of parent, grandparent, or friend the way they once did. In a nursing facility, privacy and space are at a premium. Because of the limitation of space, most of one's possessions, which provide a sense of the past, must be left behind.

> One cannot escape the institutional nature of the facility or its distance from the place, the privacy, and the possessions that residents rightfully considered part of their true home. As a patient once remarked to a researcher, "Eighty years of life packed into two boxes, a whole house reduced to half a room." (Savishinsky, 1991)

BARRIERS TO NURSING HOME ABUSE RESEARCH

Physical abuse and **psychological abuse** in nursing homes has received little research attention in spite of much anecdotal information concerning its pervasiveness. Another type of abuse that has been largely ignored in the gerontological literature is the theft of nursing home patients' possessions. To date, except for the work done by the authors, no systematic studies in this area have been conducted.

For obvious reasons, illegal and **deviant behavior** often is conducted in a covert manner. The people who engage in deviance and illegalities have a vested interest in obscuring that fact. This makes deviance difficult to study. Deviance that is committed in organizations raises even more obstacles for researchers. Except when they are the victims, organizations have a vested interest in hiding deviance that occurs within their domains. Deviance by organizational members means that the organization is not doing a good job of controlling its members, which is one of the things that organizations are supposed to do well. These general features of deviance in organizations make it an extremely difficult topic on which to gather data; this is especially true in regard to deviance in nursing homes. In a number of studies done by the authors on nursing home theft, administrators and owners were reluctant to have their employees and the families of patients participate in this type of research. Some of their objections included the following: "We are afraid it will alarm the patients and family members," "It could be detrimental to the reputation of the home," or "Why give the staff ideas?" Other reasons the administrators gave for not participating were that the staff did not have the time or they couldn't get approval from "headquarters." Often, it took numerous letters, phone calls, and visits to contact the nursing home administrators, while some were *always* "unavailable."

Some researchers believe that nursing home patients and their families are not reliable respondents for interview studies because of their fear of retaliation by the staff. After all, the same people who abuse patients are often the very ones on whom the patients depend for their care. A number of the families and patients we interviewed were reluctant to say anything unfavorable about the home or its employees. One patient, who complained bitterly about an employee stealing her candy, later changed her mind as the following case illustrates.

At a small nursing home in the Northeast, I (DH) interviewed a patient named Doris, a woman in her early seventies with a hearing deficit. As a result of her impairment, she spoke very loudly. We had very little privacy and interview conditions were less than desirable. During the course of the interview, she told me that an employee had taken a box of chocolates from her dresser drawer. She was very angry about this incident. I am certain some of the staff overheard her complaining to me about it, judging from the remarks they made to me later. At the conclusion of my visit to the home, I stopped to talk to Doris again. She told me that she was mistaken about the chocolates and to disregard what she had said earlier.

Another problem encountered in interviewing patients was obtaining informed consents from them. Some had hearing and/or speech problems, which made interviewing them extremely difficult. In addition, it was very difficult to find a private place in which to interview them, as most patients had roommates. Finally, in some homes it was simply difficult to find patients who were cognitively alert enough to interview.

In doing several survey studies, we found many cases in which nursing home administrators could not be depended upon to distribute questionnaires to their employees. Even though anonymity of the questionnaires was stressed repeatedly, many employees were still concerned that they could somehow be identified and lose their jobs.

Both the perpetrators and the victims of nursing home abuse have reasons for wishing to avoid disclosure. In addition, the managers and owners of nursing homes also have their own reasons for downplaying the seriousness of the problem. These factors, and those previously discussed, contribute to the lack of reliable information on abuse in nursing homes; they also should give us the incentive to correct this problem and to bring the dark side of the nursing home industry to light.

Chapter 2

Nursing Aides:
The Backbone of Care
in Nursing Homes

It is said that aging is not for sissies; neither is working as an aide in a nursing home. Nursing aides are the primary caregivers in these facilities. They are called the frontline workers in nursing homes because they provide an estimated 80 to 90 percent of patient care. Using data from the Current Population Survey, 1997 to 1999, Yamada (2002) summarizes the demographic characteristics and work conditions of nursing home aides (see Table 2.1). Not surprisingly, almost all the aides were female (90.1 percent). Their mean age was 36.4 years. The majority (70 percent) were white. Forty-two percent were married, and 52.2 percent had children under age eighteen. As far as education is concerned, half were high school graduates. Nursing aides had a poverty rate of 16 percent. An additional 29 percent lived near the poverty level.

WORKFORCE ISSUES AND PROBLEMS
OF NURSING HOME AIDES

Staff Turnover

Turnover rates among nursing aides are high. In fact, nursing aides have the highest turnover rates of all nursing home personnel. Their rates can reach as high as 400 percent, with an average of about 99 percent (Wunderlich et al., 1996). Some reasons for the high rate of attrition among aides include low salaries, lack of benefits, and inadequate training programs (Waxman et al., 1984). Turnover is also related to the heavy workloads of the aides. Not surprisingly, high turnover decreases the continuity and quality of care in nursing homes. It

TABLE 2.1. Demographic Characteristics of Nursing Home Aides

Characteristic	Percent
Age	
< 25	23.4
25-34	24.9
35-44	24.6
45-54	15.8
55-64	9.3
65+	2.0
Mean age	36.4
Sex	
Male	9.9
Female	90.1
Race	
White	70.6
Black	25.0
Other	4.4
Marital Status	
Married	42.8
Widowed/divorced/separated	21.9
Never married	35.3
Children	
With children under age 18	
Yes	52.2
No	47.8
Education	
Less than high school	22.6
High school graduate	49.9
Some college	23.3
4+ years of college	4.2
Income	
Personal mean income	$13,224.53
Family mean income	$33,637.57

Source: Adapted from Yamada (2002).

negatively affects the patients who do not cope well with frequent changes in staff because it tends to make their environment unpredictable. From the home's perspective, turnover results in lost productivity, replacement costs, and lowered morale among the staff.

According to a study by the Institute of Medicine (Wunderlich et al., 1996), 45 percent of nursing aides leave their jobs within the first three months, while another 30 percent leave within the first year. In her study of staff retention, Lescoe-Long (2000) offers some explanations for why aides quit after just three months of employment. These "early leavers" often find that they are unprepared for the job or that the job is different from what they had expected. Also, many feel that they are ill prepared for the types of situations and the behavioral problems they encounter with the patients. Rather than suffer through these difficulties, they decide that this is not the type of job they want, and they simply quit. Lescoe-Long (2000) further points out that:

> Aides often come from a very disadvantaged background— maybe the welfare rolls, or from a disadvantaged minority population. They want a job that is meaningful but they also want a job that pays well because they have a real need for extrinsic rewards in the workplace—finances are a major problem with them. Then they get there and find that the work isn't what they expected it to be, and the financial rewards are not that great. That's a deadly combination. They look for another job that's going to pay as well but isn't going to give as much stress. (p. 72)

Understaffing

Understaffing is a major problem of most nursing homes because it reduces the quality of care that patients receive and it increases the workload for nursing aides. Many aides try to provide good care, but due to understaffing (especially on weekends), must rush through their tasks. As a result, a significant proportion of nursing aides feel that they are pressured and overworked to the point that they cannot complete their tasks satisfactorily. "Too many patients, too little time," is a common complaint.

Henderson (1994) lists seven major tasks that day-shift nursing aides must perform and the cumulative time they consume. He notes that the tasks that are the most time-consuming are feeding, showers, and making and cleaning beds (see Table 2.2).

Bowers and Becker (1992) found that in order to survive, nursing aides cut corners out of necessity because there was not enough time to do all the work that the job required. They note that while cutting corners resulted in the breaking of rules, experienced aides knew which rules they could get away with breaking and which they could not. One of the most frequently used shortcuts for nursing aides was neglecting the patients' oral hygiene.

TABLE 2.2. Nursing Aides' Tasks and Time

Task	Cumulative hours consumed*
Patients in and out of bed	1
Food services	2.5
Making beds, cleaning beds	2.5
Shaving	1.25
Break, lunch	0.75
To and from linen/supply closet	0.25
Bathing	2.75
Miscellaneous	0.25

Source: Henderson (1994).

*Total time expended on each task by one or more nursing aides on the day shift.

A recent government study found that nine out of ten nursing homes lack an adequate number of staff. To reach the recommended staffing levels, according to a U.S. Department of Health and Human Services report, nursing homes would need to hire 81,000 to 310,000 nursing aides, making the demand for aides rise from 13 to 21 percent (Pear, 2002). According to Kayser-Jones and colleagues (2003), inadequate staffing in nursing homes has been a problem for decades:

> The recent shortage of nursing staff in all facilities, however, exacerbated the problem to a crisis level, placing an unreasonable burden on the staff who often worked double shifts several days a week. Inadequate staffing causes physical, psychological, and emotional pain to residents and their families. . . . Furthermore, the staff felt overwhelmed, overworked, and frustrated knowing that they could not provide a high standard of care. (p. 83)

Staff shortages have an even darker side, as they are also related to patient abuse. According to a patient in a nursing home: "A male nurse grabbed me, slung me on the floor, and threw me into the bed. He was in a bad mood because we were short-staffed, and he had to work two floors" (Bonnie and Wallace, 2003, p. 483).

The shortage of aides has also resulted in nursing homes having poor hiring practices and **preemployment screening procedures,** which in turn have led to a number of homes unknowingly employing workers with criminal backgrounds.

Burnout

It has been well documented that working in a nursing home is a physically demanding and emotionally challenging job that can lead to a number of work-related problems, including **burnout**. The nursing profession may be the most at risk of the helping professions for burnout due to the nature of the work, which results in high levels of job stress (Johnson, 1992). "Burnout" may be defined as physical and emotional exhaustion that results in negative feelings and indifference toward one's patients. A person suffering from burnout often feels frustrated with his or her work, and may develop feelings of guilt and failure as well as a tendency to be absent, and may eventually seek other employment. In addition, staff burnout may lead to an increased potential for abuse of patients as well as the overuse of chemical and **physical restraints** (Heine, 1986).

Research by Chappell and Novak (1992) reveals that nursing home administrators can help alleviate the effects of burnout and job stress on nursing aides by decreasing or changing their workloads as well as providing them with rewards on the job. In addition, they suggest training for nursing aides to help them in dealing with cognitively impaired patients.

Training

Nursing aides, as we have noted, compose the largest proportion of caregiving workers in nursing homes and provide most of the hands-on care, yet they often receive inadequate training. Since the passage of the Nursing Home Reform Act in the **Omnibus Budget Reconciliation Act** (OBRA 1987), nursing aides are required to have a minimum of seventy-five hours of formal training and to pass a competency examination within four months of being employed. In addition, they also must have twelve hours of in-service training per year. According to federal law, each state must maintain a **nursing aides' registry** of all individuals who have satisfactorily completed an approved nursing aide training program in that state.

In spite of these requirements for certification, it is well-known that many aides are still inadequately trained for their duties. Although new staff receive training on the physical needs of patients, they often are not trained to handle interpersonal issues. For example, many types of behavior problems that aides encounter, such as noncompliance and aggression, are difficult to manage. It is important to help aides learn and practice strategies to deal with these conflictual situations.

It is not uncommon for nursing aides to report patients' tendency to act physically and psychologically aggressive toward them. For instance, Goodridge and colleagues (1996) administered a questionnaire to 126 nursing aides in a 320-bed Canadian nursing home. Physical aggression from patients during the past month was reported by about 70 percent of the nursing aides. The most common types of abuse were being pushed, grabbed, shoved, or pinched by the patients. Eighty-four percent of the aides reported incidents of psychological aggression from patients in the past month, such as being insulted, threatened, or sworn at. Studies reveal that abuse of aides tends to most frequently occur while the aides are assisting the patients with self-care (Newbern, 1987; Goodridge et al., 1996). In a nursing home that one of the authors visited, she overheard a conversation between two nursing aides. One of the aides held up her arms and said, "Just look at these scratches. So help me, I'll never give that woman a bath again." Attempting to control the patients' aggressive behavior is a difficult problem for the staff, especially when a situation becomes violent. Such behavior can injure the aide and the patient.

A number of studies have implicated physical and psychological aggression by patients toward caregivers as a major factor that increases the risk of abusive behavior toward patients. For example, Newbern (1987) found that aggressive patients were four times as likely to be abused as were compliant and passive patients. The aides' response to psychological and physical abuse may be compassion and understanding or, for some, it may be retaliation, such as stealing patients' possessions or physically maltreating them. When patients violate the expectations of proper patient behavior, this may unfortunately have the effect of temporarily releasing aides from the restraining power of the **norm** that prohibits patient abuse (Stannard, 1973). Focus group interviews with nursing aides revealed that many of the aides felt that rough treatment of a patient who was physically aggressive with them was justified and not abusive. After all, they had a right to protect themselves from injury (Bonnie and Wallace, 2003).

Besides being abused by patients, nursing home personnel, especially aides, are also physically abused by patients' family members. Vinton and Mazza (1994), in an exploratory survey of seventy Florida nursing homes, found that over a six-month period personnel of the nursing homes reported thirteen cases of physical aggression by family members. The most frequently cited issues for contention by the family members (primarily spouses and children) were how the specific care needs of their relatives were being met, followed by the overall quality of their care, and the theft of their relatives' possessions.

Nursing aides do not have halos *or* horns. As Foner (1994) noted in the home that she studied, "The aides are neither saints nor monsters but fall somewhere in between. Only a small minority are consistently cruel or consistently warm and supportive" (p. 38).

The Environment

Tellis-Nyak and Tellis-Nyak (1989) described the vicious cycle of staff discontent and poor patient care that occurs in many nursing homes.

> In too many nursing homes the institutional culture prevails. Within it aides are only hired hands; no one provides for their affective needs nor cares if it alienates them. And being in the constant company of dependent elderly residents, the aides begin to individualize their problems. They make their wards the ready targets of their discontent and resentment.
>
> And that completes the vicious cycle. Two parties, both powerless, little respected, and hardly recognized by society are made to face each other in a difficult setting not of their own making. They are bound in an intimate association, but enjoy little intimacy. Neither party controls the institutional environment in which they exist, neither can break the negative cycle, and so the problem feeds on itself. (p. 312)

The Working Environment of Nursing Aides

Low wages and poor benefits, compounded by the emotional and physical strain of the work, the physical and/or social isolation from professionals and sometimes peers, the lack of sufficient organizational training and support, and the absence of opportunities for advancement have all been cited as factors contributing to difficulties in recruiting frontline workers, to high turnover, and to quality problems in long-term care. (Feldman, 1994, p. 7)

NARRATIVES OF NURSING HOME AIDES

As part of our preparation for writing this book, we interviewed nursing aides in a number of different homes. These interviews provided us with a deeper understanding and greater appreciation for the difficult and complex work that aides do every day. By and large, the views expressed by the aides mirrored what other researchers have found. A recurring theme throughout the interviews was how important it was to be appreciated. Most of the nursing aides said that they liked to help others and their work made them feel that they were doing something worthwhile. For example, when asked what the best thing was about working in a nursing home, an aide said:

> The thanks I get are few. But this one lady that I take care of, I always get a nice thank-you from her and her family and that means a lot to me. I would say that it's just once in a blue moon you will get a thank you, and it's like, well, that was worth it, and I keep going.

Some aides said they liked working in a nursing home because they enjoy being around older persons and the patients are like family to them.

> I like working with the elderly because I remember when I was growing up my grandmother was very ill and my mom took care of her. It makes me feel good if I can help the elderly. I have a lot of respect for the older population and I like to see their later years nice and happy and that they are well taken care of.

In answer to the question, "What is it like to work in a nursing home?" one aide said:

> It is challenging and interesting. It is also frustrating and annoying. Sometimes it is depressing and sometimes it is very uplifting but it is never the same. . . . You have to know when to take time out. I have walked away from a lot of people. I did it the other day. I thought it wise to shut my mouth and not say a word. It may be rude to walk away, but it's going to be ruder if you don't.

Finally, according to one aide: "The work is physically demanding, there's a lot of lifting, and you are on your feet for long hours, but the work is very satisfying and rewarding."

Chapter 3

Understanding Abuse

Many terms, from "granny bashing" to "the battered elder syndrome," have been used to describe the physical maltreatment of older persons. Today "elder abuse" is the most widely used expression, but its meaning has been broadened to encompass nonphysical forms of maltreatment, including psychological abuse and property or **material abuse**. Physical abuse refers to acts that inflict physical pain or injury on nursing home patients, such as hitting or slapping a patient or the inappropriate use of physical restraints. Psychological abuse includes acts that cause patients to experience emotional pain or fear, such as calling them degrading names or otherwise verbally abusing or threatening them. Finally, material abuse is defined as the theft or misuse of a patient's possessions or financial resources.

Criminologists, gerontologists, and others interested in the problems of nursing home patients have developed a number of different theories and perspectives to explain abuse in nursing homes. Some theories focus on the offenders; others note the special characteristics of the elderly as potential victims; and still others direct attention to the nursing home environment itself as an important causal factor in abuse. However, at present no single theory is sufficient to provide a completely satisfactory explanation of any type of elder abuse. In this chapter, we review contemporary research on abuse in nursing homes and attempt to synthesize what is known into a coherent understanding of the problem of mistreatment in nursing homes. We begin by adopting a criminological perspective on elder abuse. We show how criminological theory can be applied to this problem.

WHY NURSING HOMES MAY BE GOOD FOR ABUSERS

When most of us contemplate crime problems, we think about criminals. We want to know why do they do it and how can we stop them. Focusing on offenders is natural, but it is not necessarily the best way to think about crime. In the late 1970s, two sociologists at the University of Illinois developed an important and widely influential new theory of crime. The approach developed by Lawrence Cohen and Marcus Felson (1979) has subsequently come to be known as **routine activity,** or *opportunity theory.* It provides a useful conceptual framework for helping to understand nursing home abuse from a criminological perspective.

According to Cohen and Felson, in order for a crime to occur three things have to happen at the same time and place. These are called the *elements of crime.* First, there must be a *motivated offender*—a person or persons with criminal inclinations and the ability to carry out those inclinations. Second, there must be some person or object that is the target of the offender's criminal actions. Criminologists call this person or object the *suitable target.* Third, the target must not be adequately guarded or protected. In criminological terms, this is called a *lack of capable guardianship.* When these three elements of crime occur at the same time and place—that is, the presence of a motivated offender, a suitable target, and the absence of capable guardianship—then some sort of crime is very likely to occur. This theory recognizes that deviance and crime depend not only on the motivations of criminals but also on the opportunities they encounter.

What makes a target suitable for crime depends on whether the target is a material object or a person. When the target is some sort of object or piece of property, suitability is determined by the value of the object, its portability, and its accessibility. Items that are valuable, easy to carry or conceal, and easy to obtain make more attractive targets for thieves than those that are not very valuable or difficult to move. Obviously, for most thieves, a nice diamond ring left unattended on a nightstand in a patient's room is a far more fetching target than a refrigerator in a locked house. When a criminal wants to attack a person, then suitability is determined by the person's vulnerability or their ability to protect themselves. Someone who is armed to the teeth makes a less attractive target for assault or robbery than someone who is frail and weak.

For a variety of reasons, some nursing homes provide an ideal setting for the elements of crime to converge. They bring together motivated offenders and suitable targets under conditions of low or nonexistent guardianship. Thus, it is not surprising that crime and abuse are no strangers to nursing homes. From a criminological perspective, it follows almost automatically from the organizational structure and the nature of the people and work in nursing homes. In the following sections, we consider each of the three elements of crime in relation to nursing homes and their patients.

NURSING HOMES AND THE MOTIVATED OFFENDER

Caregiver Stress

Many motivated offenders can be found in nursing homes because of the stress, hard work, and low pay found in many facilities. Nursing aides, those who work most directly and most often with patients, are at greatest risk of becoming stressed. Working directly with patients can be difficult. Patients often can be demanding or irritating. This can lead to caregiver stress, which research has shown to be one of the primary factors in physical and psychological abuse of patients.

A study by Pillemer and Moore (1989) that was based on telephone interviews with nursing home staff found a number of stress-related factors that tend to be predictors of physical and psychological abuse of patients by the staff. These stress-related factors include job dissatisfaction, viewing the patients as children, burnout, and conflicts with patients. Stress and conflict with patients can also lead to other forms of abuse, such as theft. Harris and Benson (1999) surveyed staff members in nursing homes and found that employees who stole from patients reported more conflict with them than did nonthieves.

Nursing home workers frequently react to stress at work by abusing the patients to whom they provide care:

Staff members who receive low wages, whose working conditions are poor, who are employed in "dead-end" jobs, and who work under overly demanding supervisors and indifferent administrators are the people who are considered most likely to abuse residents. These staff members sometimes describe the residents under their care as overly demanding and ungrateful for the care they receive. The nature of the caregiving work with institutionalized elderly populations, which comprise elderly people with numerous impairments, including Alzheimer's disease, may cause low morale, high rates of staff "burnout" and turnover, and inadequate care of residents, including abuse. (Kosberg and Nahmiash, 1996, p. 40)

Another factor that also may be associated with the stressful working conditions of nursing aides is racial conflict, demonstrated specifically by racial slurs and stereotyping. Some nursing aides who perceive that patients are prejudiced toward them because of their race feel that patients think they do not do a good job or unfairly accuse them of things they did not do (Noelker and Harel, 2001). This situation may result in negative interactions between aides and patients and can lead to patient abuse.

Job Dissatisfaction and Unfairness

In addition to stress, staff members who are potential offenders may find motivation from other sources. Nursing home workers, similar to workers everywhere, want to be treated fairly. When workers think they are not being treated fairly, this can in some instances motivate deviant and criminal behavior in the workplace. A large body of research on workers in organizations documents that when workers feel they are being treated unfairly this leads to feelings of resentment and to efforts to get even. People who work for organizations expect to receive rewards in return for high-quality job performance. For example, if people perform well and they receive high pay levels, this would be considered a **fair ratio**. However, if they performed well but received a low pay level, this would be considered an unfair ratio and might motivate the workers to take action. While feelings of unfairness in the workplace are not unique to nursing homes or to nursing home workers, the outcomes from them may be substantially more serious. In nursing homes, workers who are dissatisfied with their jobs or filled with resentment over perceived unfair treatment may take out their frustrations on patients.

A significant proportion of nursing home employees are poorly paid (particularly those in non-skilled positions, such as nursing aides, housekeepers, and laundry staff) (Waxman et al., 1984). The meager financial rewards received by some nursing home employees may motivate them to supplement their pay through theft. Although it is difficult to determine whether nursing home workers are any more likely than other types of workers to feel that they are treated unfairly, evidence that most nursing aides feel that they have to work too hard for the low pay they receive exists. In a questionnaire administered to nursing home aides about their job situation, nearly all the respondents wrote they were overworked and underpaid (Harris and Benson, 1997). Given the minimum wages that they receive and the stressful and physically taxing work they do, it is not surprising that most nursing aides think that the system is unfair and unjust. The reaction of some of these employees to this perceived injustice may be to steal from the patients "to even up the score." In this way, they may feel that they are doing something to resolve some of the inequities they perceive in the workplace.

Low Self-Control

Another prominent criminological theory also may be applied to the problem of abuse in nursing homes. This **general theory of crime,** developed by Gottfredson and Hirschi (1990), is based on the idea that people who hurt and take advantage of others have low self-control. Individuals with low self-control are impulsive, risk-taking, self-centered, and shortsighted people. They are easily provoked and take advantage of criminal opportunities whenever and wherever they find them. This theory does not assume that offenders are motivated by such factors as stress or unfairness. However, it assumes that offenders need no special motivation to commit their offenses. Rather, they commit offenses because of low self-control. With respect to offenses such as physical abuse and theft in nursing homes, according to this theory, the personal characteristics of some people who work in nursing homes, rather than the stressful work they perform, may be the most important cause of their abusive behavior.

Individuals with low self-control have many other problems besides their propensity to engage in criminal and deviant behavior. They tend to do poorly in school and have difficulty finding and keeping good jobs. When they do seek work, they tend to gravitate toward employment in low-skill and low-wage positions. Unfortunately, many entry-level jobs in nursing homes, such as the positions of nursing aide, janitor, food service worker, and laundry worker are such low-skill and low-wage positions. Individuals with higher levels of education and skills and more likely higher levels of self-control often are unwilling to accept or stay in such positions. They expect something better. Hence, when making staffing and hiring decisions, nursing home administrators likely have to choose from a less-than-ideal pool of job applicants. Of course, it is not true that most of the people who work in nursing homes are criminal or deviant or have low self-control. The majority of workers are honest and caring individuals who do the best that they can in the difficult and important work that nursing homes do. Nor is it the case that nursing homes are the only places that people with low self-control can find work. Any industry that relies on low-skill and low-wage workers will tend to attract the same sort of individuals. Nevertheless, it is important to acknowledge that the *proportion* of employees in nursing homes that has low self-control is likely to be higher than the proportion of employees in more lucrative and less stressful lines of work.

Thus, for a variety of reasons—stressful work, low pay, racial conflict, unpleasant working conditions, and the personal characteristics of some of the individuals who end up working in nursing homes—nursing homes may have more than their fair share of people who are motivated to engage in some form of abusive behavior toward patients. This is the first of the three necessary elements for crime to take place.

PATIENTS AND THEIR POSSESSIONS
AS SUITABLE TARGETS

For someone who is motivated to inflict physical or psychological abuse, patients in nursing homes make ideal targets. They are highly vulnerable. According to Ansello (1996), "the characteristics of the elderly person, specifically, incapacities and impairments, render the elderly person frail and vulnerable. This vulnerability may predispose them to exploitation by a second party" (p. 20). Elderly patients are unlikely to be able to defend themselves physically. In addition, because the elderly often are frail, impaired, and dependent on others, they may be perceived as belonging to a socially stigmatized category—useless, nonproductive, and possessing little social value. As a result, some people may believe that victimizing them is less serious and less important than victimizing individuals who make more productive contributions to society.

Patients in nursing homes also make good targets for those who wish to steal. Patients often want to keep personal items, such as jewelry, money, and clothing, in their rooms. Small, easy to conceal, and relatively valuable, these items make attractive targets for thieves. Also helpful to potential thieves are the physical impairments and cognitive disabilities from which many patients suffer. Because of these conditions, patients may lack the ability to keep track of their personal belongings. Most patients (78 percent) in nursing homes require help in taking care of their personal possessions, and just as many need assistance in securing their possessions (Dey, 1997). In addition, if patients are mentally incompetent, employees may feel that theft from them is not as morally wrong as it would be from those who are aware of and appreciate their personal property. A suitable target is the second of the three necessary elements for crime to take place.

GUARDIANSHIP IN NURSING HOMES

Guardianship refers to how well a person or object is protected. Individuals who do not live in nursing homes can take many steps to guard or protect themselves and their possessions. They can lock their doors, subscribe to home security services, keep watchdogs, and even buy firearms for self-defense. They can exert control over the people they let into their homes or that they come in contact with when they leave their homes. They can avoid places where criminals are known to congregate. Patients in nursing homes, however, often are less able to employ these commonsense methods of protecting themselves and their possessions. For public opinion on this subject, see Exhibit 3.1.

For obvious reasons, patients cannot lock their doors or deny access to their rooms to nursing home staff, nor can they install a burglar alarm or keep a gun under their pillow. They often are unable to block access to their persons or their possessions. When it comes to guardianship, however, the biggest problem that patients face is that the very nature of nursing homes requires them to continually be in close proximity with potential motivated offenders. As part of their work, nursing aides as well as housekeepers and other employees must visit patients' rooms on a regular basis, at times when the patient is absent, asleep, or otherwise incapacitated. Hence, nursing home workers have easy access to patients' possessions. Staff members also have physical access to patients, helping them to feed themselves, get dressed, bathe, engage in physical therapy, and move about the home. All of these points of contact between the staff member and the patient are potential points at which disputes between the two may arise. These disputes might eventually lead to abuse. Indeed, nearly any time that staff members have access to patients, provides opportunity for physical or psychological abuse.

EXHIBIT 3.1. Survey Question Addressed to General Public

Do you think the following is something that happens to almost all nursing home residents, many of them, some, or hardly any?

Residents can rely on their personal belongings being safe.

Almost all	Many	Some	Hardly any
16%	15%	34%	30%

Source: The NewsHour with Jim Lehrer/Kaiser Family Foundation/Harvard School of Public Health National Survey on Nursing Homes, October 2001.

To summarize, because of the nature of the work and the economics of the industry, nursing homes are places in which motivated offenders are likely to have access to suitable targets under conditions of low or nonexistent guardianship (the third element necessary for crime to take place). Because of their dependency and physical and mental impairments, many patients are easy prey for those who wish to mistreat them. At the same time, "their possessions also make suitable targets for thieves who can operate in a nursing home with the ease of a fox in a henhouse" (Sinclair, 1990). The elements of crime are in place and the formula for abuse is now complete.

COUNTERVAILING FORCES

Sinclair's imagery of a "fox in a henhouse" is compelling, but it is an exaggeration. Nursing home patients are not completely unprotected; nor are they completely at the mercy of ruthless employees. Protecting patients, standing between them and harm, is (or at least should be) the nursing home administration. Administrators have the ability and the duty to supervise employees and discipline or terminate those who engage in misconduct. The issue here is how rigorously and effectively they can carry out these tasks. As with many aspects of organizational functioning, it is likely that nursing homes and their administrators vary dramatically in these abilities.

Because elder abuse in nursing homes takes place within an organizational setting, it is important to consider what we call the organization's deterrence environment. The deterrence environment refers to the perceived certainty of detection and perceived severity of punishment among those who are in a position to commit offenses within an organization. When perceived certainty and severity are high, the deterrence environment is strong and offending rates within the organization should be low. Unfortunately, similar to other organizations, nursing home administrations may not be very effective at detecting misconduct and therefore may not have a very strong deterrence environment (Hollinger and Clark, 1983). Even when misconduct is detected in organizations, administrators often are loath to discipline their employees. For a variety of reasons, organizations may prefer to ignore employee misconduct if it is not too serious or to treat it informally rather than involving law enforcement officials. For example, many employers tolerate a small amount of misappropriation or misuse of company materials, such as office supplies, because policing the whereabouts of every pen and pencil is inefficient. Taking a pen or pad of paper for personal use is treated as a minor benefit. When employees commit more serious offenses against their employers, the response often is to fire them but not to report the matter to the police. Involving the police is time-consuming for administrative staff, may lower employee morale, and may reflect poorly on the organization in the eyes of its clients or customers. Thus, in many organizations the certainty and severity of punishment for misconduct is low. Nursing homes are no different than other organizations in this regard. The problem of how to control employees is a never-ending one.

SUMMARY

Taking a criminological perspective on the problem of elder abuse in nursing homes is helpful. It permits us to bring together disparate lines of research into a cohesive whole. The routine activities perspective clearly demonstrates that to attack the problem of abuse in nursing homes, we will have to operate on multiple levels. It is not enough to call for harsher penalties for those convicted of abusing patients in nursing homes. Offenders are only one piece of the puzzle. In addition to offenders and their motivations, we must also consider target suitability and guardianship. Reducing target suitability and improving guardianship may be just as important as punishing offenders in addressing and alleviating the problem of maltreatment in nursing homes.

PART II:
NURSING HOME THEFT

Chapter 4

Employees and Theft

As we noted in Chapter 1, investigating misconduct in nursing homes is difficult. Many barriers stand in the way of researchers. Most important is the understandable reluctance of nursing home administrators to cooperate in studies that may uncover information that reflects poorly on their facilities. Even when administrators are willing to participate, employees and other staff members still may be hesitant about participating, especially if they are asked to provide information on work-related misconduct by themselves or their colleagues.

These obstacles are real and significant, but they are not unique to nursing homes. Criminologists who study white-collar and corporate crime long have known that studying deviance in organizational settings poses special problems (Hollinger and Clark, 1983). In all formal organizations, the people in charge strive to protect the reputation and integrity of the businesses they lead by limiting the flow of unflattering information. Likewise, employees are expected to be loyal and to try to keep the organization's "dirty laundry" in-house. For these and other reasons, we are limited in what we can learn about crime and deviance within work organizations.

The difficulties of studying crime and deviance in organizations, however, should not dissuade us from attempting to gather as much empirical information as we can. Criminologists and social scientists have developed techniques for studying deviance in organizations that, although not foolproof, are nevertheless a vast improvement over armchair conjectures and anecdotal evidence. In this chapter and the one that follows, we report on the results of the study that we have conducted on nursing homes using these techniques. (A complete description of the methodologies used in our study is found in the Appendix.)

RESULTS FROM THE SURVEY OF EMPLOYEES

We surveyed 1,116 employees in forty-seven nursing homes. Although this is a relatively large sample of employees, it is not necessarily perfectly representative of all of the employees in the nursing homes we studied. We conservatively estimate that approximately 22 percent of the employees responded to our questionnaire. Although this response rate is lower than ideal, it is quite similar to response rates reported by other nursing home researchers (e.g., Goergen, 2001). It is important to keep in mind that a questionnaire on such a sensitive topic as employee theft may threaten some employees, who may refuse to participate out of fear of exposure. Overall, we were not surprised at our response rate because in other smaller pilot studies that we had conducted we received a similar response (Harris and Benson, 1997).

Characteristics of the People Who Work in Nursing Homes

Table 4.1 provides descriptive information about the sample of employees. The sample is overwhelmingly female (89 percent) and white (81 percent). More than half of the sample is married (57 percent), and more than two-thirds have at least a high school diploma. The average age is just over forty, and half of the sample has an annual household income of less than $30,000. Overall, the sample could be described as consisting primarily of middle- to lower-middle-class individuals. The typical person in the sample is a married, middle-aged white woman of moderate means who has a high school education.

Because occupational position is related to opportunities to steal from patients, we include information on it in Table 4.2. As shown there, the distribution of job titles indicates that nursing aides were the most common respondents to our survey. This result is not surprising, because nationally, aides represent about 45 percent of all nursing home employees (Strahan, 1997). Even though nursing aides represent the modal category in our sample, they are nevertheless underrepresented. They constitute only 29.7 percent of our sample (30.1 percent of those who answered this question). Although aides

TABLE 4.1. Characteristics of the Sample of Employees

Characteristic	Percent or mean
Sex	
Female	89.3
Male	10.6
Race	
White	81.0
Black	11.4
Mexican American/Hispanic	3.2
Other	4.4
Marital Status	
Married	57.1
Widowed	5.4
Divorced	10.8
Separated	3.7
Cohabiting	5.3
Never married	17.8
Education	
Junior high or less	1.9
Some high school	6.7
High school diploma	24.7
Some college	26.3
Business or trade	19.2
College degree	13.0
Postgraduate	8.2
Total Household Income	
Less than $10,000	9.1
$10,001 to $20,000	22.8
$20,001 to $30,000	18.2
$30,001 to $40,000	15.7
$40,001 to $50,000	11.2
More than $50,000	23.1
Age	40.7

are underrepresented, the demographic profile of our sample of aides mirrors results reported in other studies of nursing aides (Bowers and Becker, 1992; Chappell and Novak, 1992).

The aides in our sample are overwhelmingly female (94.2 percent). Most are white (75.5 percent), and the mean age is 36.8. About half of the aides (48.1 percent) are married, and nearly half have no schooling beyond high school (48.9 percent). Nurses (including RNs

TABLE 4.2. Job Titles of the Employee Sample

Job title	Frequency	Percent
Registered Nurse	148	13.5
LPN	124	11.3
Nursing Aide	331	30.1
Housekeeper	64	5.8
Laundry Worker	23	2.1
Therapist	42	3.8
Office Worker	88	8.0
Food Service Worker	101	9.2
Social Worker	33	3.0
Maintenance Worker	16	1.5
Administrator	26	2.4
Other	102	9.3
Total	1,098	100

and LPNs) constitute the next most frequent category in the sample at just under 25 percent. It is important to note that over half of the employee respondents (55.9 percent) are directly involved in caring for patients. Other job titles that probably are closely involved with patients include "therapist" (3.4 percent) and "social worker" (2.9 percent). Among the support staff, housekeepers (6.0 percent), laundry workers (2.2 percent), and food service workers (8.7 percent) make up approximately 17 percent of the sample. Office workers, maintenance, administrators, and others make up the remaining 20 percent of the sample. Some of the respondents in the "other" category probably work directly with patients, such as activity assistants and recreational assistants.

A substantial majority of the respondents were experienced nursing home workers, meaning that they reported working in the present home or another home for more than one year. Over one-third (35.5 percent) of the sample said they had worked in their present home for more than five years. About one-quarter (27.4 percent), on the other hand, had worked in the present home for less than one year, but most of these individuals had worked elsewhere in the nursing home industry for longer periods. In sum, most respondents have had substantial time to observe or participate in theft from patients.

On the basis of routine activity theory (see Chapter 3), we assumed that access to patients' rooms is a prerequisite of theft. Hence, we asked respondents about how often, if ever, they enter patients' rooms and whether they typically work alone or with others. We hoped with these questions to better identify who has the greatest opportunities to steal from patients. The responses indicate that the vast majority of nursing home employees at least have some opportunity to commit theft from patients. Almost nine out of ten (86.9 percent) reported going into patients' rooms at least once or twice a week. Eighty percent visit patients' rooms at least once or twice a day, and fully two-thirds go in many times a day. The percentage of people who report frequently going into patients' rooms is greater than the percentage of people in direct care positions, which means that other individuals besides nurses and nursing aides have opportunities for theft. Most of the respondents said that they usually work with another person close by (68.3 percent). Less than 10 percent said they usually work alone.

Employees Who Steal from Patients

Only seventeen employees reported that they had taken something from a patient, making the theft rate 1.53 percent. This rate is about half of that observed in an earlier smaller study that we conducted. That project involved only six nursing homes in the southeast region of the United States and a total of 281 respondents, of whom eleven (3.9 percent) self-reported theft from patients (Harris and Benson, 1997). The low rate found in the national survey may have resulted from the underrepresentation of nursing aides in the sample. Interestingly, of the seventeen who reported taking things from patients, a majority (eleven) said they had done so on more than one occasion. However, for reasons that we will soon discuss, we believe that this rate probably underestimates to some unknown extent the true rate of employee theft in nursing homes.

Because of the low rate of self-reported theft, it is difficult to find factors that will reliably distinguish employees who are more likely to steal from those who refrain from theft. Nevertheless, we can get a general idea of who these people are and what they steal from patients. Table 4.3 presents a comparison between those who self-reported theft versus those who did not on selected sociodemographic characteristics. The rates of self-reported theft are nearly equal for males and females and for whites and African Americans. Some evidence suggests that marital status is related to theft, as those who are cohabiting or who have never been married have slightly elevated levels of theft compared to those who are married or who have been married in the past.

TABLE 4.3. Characteristics of Self-Reported Thieves and Non-Thieves

Characteristic	Self-reported theft	
	Yes	No
Age (Mean)	37.5	40.7
Sex		
Female	1.5% (15)	98.5% (962)
Male	1.7% (2)	98.3% (114)
Race		
White	1.4% (12)	98.6% (867)
Black	1.6% (2)	98.4% (122)
Others	0.0% (0)	100% (82)
Marital Status		
Married	1.5% (9)	98.5% (611)
Cohabiting	3.4% (2)	96.6% (56)
Widowed, divorced, or separated	0.9% (2)	98.0% (213)
Never married	2.1% (3)	99.1% (190)
Education		
Less than high school	0.0% (0)	100% (93)
High school diploma	1.5% (4)	98.5% (262)
Some college	3.1% (9)	96.9% (278)
Technical school	0.5% (1)	99.5% (209)
College degree	2.1% (3)	97.9% (140)
Advanced study	0.0% (0)	100% (89)
Income		
Less than $10,000	0.0% (0)	100% (96)
$10,001 to $20,000	2.1% (5)	97.9% (236)
$20,001 to $30,000	1.0% (2)	99.0% (191)
$30,001 to $40,000	1.8% (3)	98.2% (164)
$40,001 to $50,000	2.5% (3)	97.5% (116)
More than $50,000	1.6% (4)	98.4% (240)

Surprisingly, the findings on education and income show slightly higher levels of theft among the more educated and well-to-do than their less educated and well-off counterparts. However, all of these results must be interpreted cautiously, as the numbers of self-reported thefts in these sociodemographic categories are very small and may reflect only differences in reporting. For example, more educated and well-to-do respondents may have more experience filling out questionnaires and with research techniques designed to protect confidentiality of responses. Hence, they may be more willing to trust our assurances regarding confidentiality and to respond truthfully than less educated respondents to our sensitive, personal questions.

The Social Psychology of Theft from Patients

In regard to age, race, and sex, those who self-reported theft do not appear to be distinguishable sociodemographically from those who did not report theft. This result indicates that we need to look elsewhere to understand why employees take the possessions of patients. As we noted in Chapter 2, many of the theories that have been proposed to explain employee abuse and mistreatment of patients attribute theft to the stressful nature of work in nursing homes. Dealing with patients is difficult work—work that is often not very well remunerated. Although patients often are frail and dependent, they also can be both physically and verbally abusive to the staff members who have to deal directly with them on a daily basis. It is not surprising that the demands of the job sometimes lead to caregiver stress and burnout and to unsympathetic attitudes toward patients. Neither would it be surprising for staff members who have been abused by patients to develop feelings of anger and resentment toward patients. These feelings in turn could serve as motivations for theft from patients. In addition, it is reasonable to assume that levels of job satisfaction in general may have a correlation with theft. Employees who feel dissatisfied with their work because of its demeaning or thankless nature or who feel anger toward the nursing home because of overwork, low pay, or dictatorial behavior by supervisors may feel less constrained about hurting patients than employees who enjoy their jobs. To explore these possibilities, we asked the staff members a series of questions about their attitudes toward patients, their experiences with them, and their general level of job satisfaction.

To help us understand how employees feel about patients, we asked the employees to tell us how much they agreed or disagreed with a series of eleven statements describing their attitudes toward them. Some of the statements were positively worded, as in, for example, "I treat patients as if they are family" and "Patients come first, no matter what." Other statements were negatively worded, as in "Most patients are more trouble than they are worth" and "I don't like listening to patients talk about their problems." The four response categories ranged from "strongly agree" to "strongly disagree," and a fifth category, "does not apply," was available for employees who had no direct contact with patients. After reversing the coding on some of the items so that high numbers reflected positive feelings about patients, we combined the eleven items into an index of "attitudes toward patients."

We used the same approach to measure job satisfaction in general and attitudes toward supervisors. Employees were asked to indicate how strongly they agreed or disagreed with a series of statements about their jobs, such as "I dislike my work," "Most of the time I feel good about how I do my job," and "My job means more to me than just money." The items about supervisors included such statements as "When I do a good job, my supervisors show their appreciation" and "My supervisors don't appreciate the physical and emotional strain of my job." As with our questions on attitudes toward patients, some of the items reflected positive job satisfaction or feelings about supervisors while others were negatively worded. After recoding the answers so that high scores reflected high job satisfaction and positive attitudes toward supervisors, we summed the respective groups of items to form two indexes: "job satisfaction" and "attitudes toward supervisors."

Measuring abuse by patients toward employees required a slightly different approach. Rather than asking employees to agree or disagree with statements, we asked them to tell us how often they experienced negative interactions with patients. Employees were asked to indicate how often patients "start arguments with you," "verbally abuse you (for example, they yell, insult, or swear at you)" and "physically abuse you (for example, they push, grab, hit, or scratch you)."

The five response categories ranged from "never or practically never" to "every day." We added together the responses to these three items to form an index of "maltreatment by patients."

By comparing the mean index scores of those who self-reported theft to those who did not report theft, we learned that the former have more negative attitudes toward patients and are more likely to experience mistreatment from patients (see Table 4.4). For the self-reported thieves, the mean score on the index of maltreatment by patients was 9.12, compared to 6.44 for those who did not report theft. This difference is statistically significant at the .01 level, meaning it is highly unlikely to have resulted from pure chance or measurement error. Self-reported thieves also have less positive attitudes toward patients as indicated by their mean score of 34.06 versus the mean score of 36.87 for the non-thieves on the index. This difference is also statistically significant. Finally, the self-reported thieves have lower job satisfaction and less positive attitudes toward supervisors than non-thieves, but these differences are not large enough to be statistically significant.

Taken together, these findings suggest that several sources of motivation for theft from patients might exist. Employees may take items from patients out of a desire for revenge because of what they interpret as mistreatment from patients. If not out of a sense of revenge, then theft may arise out of a general dislike of patients or a lack of sympathy toward them. Most of us are socialized to feel that it is

TABLE 4.4. Attitudes Toward Patients and Work

	Mean Score	
Index	Thieves	Non-thieves
Attitudes toward patients[a]	34.06*	36.87
Attitudes toward supervisors[a]	24.09	25.91
Job satisfaction[a]	55.58	57.49
Maltreatment by patients[b]	9.12*	6.44

a High scores for the first three indexes indicate more positive feelings.

b High scores for the maltreatment index indicate more frequent mistreatment by patients toward employee.

* $p < .01$

wrong to hurt others unnecessarily, and we feel guilty when we do so. The greater potential that we have to experience these feelings, the more we are held back from engaging in untoward actions, because we wish to avoid feeling guilty and bad about ourselves. Indeed, one prominent theory of crime assumes that a major difference between criminal offenders and law-abiding people is that the former population has a reduced ability to feel sympathy for others (Gottfredson and Hirschi, 1990). If we do not care about the other person, or if we actively dislike someone, then we are less likely to empathize with him or her or to feel guilty about hurting him or her. That those who steal have more negative attitudes toward patients than those who do not may indicate that the former are less likely to feel empathy for patients, and hence less likely to worry about the harm that their actions cause patients. Thus, they are freer to commit theft without feeling guilty. Finally, the lower levels of job satisfaction among the thieves may indicate that poor working conditions or the perception of poor working conditions may motivate theft among employees.

Opportunity and Organizational Location of Thieves

All crimes require that the offender have access to the target, which can be either a person or some form of property. Because of the nature of their service, nursing homes provide potential offenders with specialized access to the property of victims. Employees in nursing homes (and, for that matter, other institutions that manage, service, or care for people for extended periods of time—such as hospitals, prisons, hotels, and rehabilitation facilities) often have legitimate access to other people's rooms and hence their possessions. Hospital personnel must check on their charges, clean rooms, and deliver medications. These duties as well as others provide reasons for entering private rooms. Maids go into hotel rooms when the guests are out but their belongings are not. In nursing homes, aides and nurses routinely go into patients' rooms when patients are not present, or when they are asleep or otherwise incapacitated. When nursing home personnel are in patients' rooms, they have access to property. The work routines of some personnel require them to go into patients' rooms more often than others. Thus, it is reasonable to assume that some nursing home personnel have greater opportunities for theft than others.

To explore how access to patients' rooms is related to theft, we asked the employees how often they went into patients' rooms as part of their jobs. The response categories were "never or almost never," "once or twice a week," "once or twice a day," and "many times a day." We also asked how often ("usually," "occasionally," or "usually not") the employee worked with another employee close by. Our reasoning behind this question was that the presence of others would usually act as a deterrent to theft, unless, of course, two or more employees form a conspiracy to commit theft together.

Not surprisingly, given the makeup of the sample, a large majority of the respondents go into patients' rooms many times during a typical workday, and they usually work with another person close by. Two-thirds of the respondents said that as part of their jobs they went into patients' rooms many times a day, and two-thirds also said that they usually work with another person close by. Also, as expected, nursing aides were the persons most likely to go into patients' rooms often. Over 90 percent of the aides said that they went into rooms many times a day. However, contrary to our expectations, employees who reported greater access to patients' rooms and working alone were not more likely to steal from patients than employees who reported less access. This result appears to undermine the routine activities perspective on theft but, for reasons that we will make clearer in the next section, we should not jump to that conclusion. As we will show, observations of theft are strongly related to access to patients' rooms. For now, however, it appears that the social psychological variables that we have just discussed are more important in distinguishing thieves from non-thieves than are occupational work routines.

Perceived Risks and Theft

The rational choice approach to crime assumes that potential offenders are interested in avoiding punishment and that the perceived risk of punishment is an important factor in criminal decision making. Presumably, people who believe in a high likelihood that they will get caught if they do something wrong and who think that something bad will happen to them if they are caught are less likely to steal than people who think they can get away with theft and who think that little is likely to happen even if they are caught. The likelihood of getting caught and punished as a result of theft deters some nursing home workers. To see how perceived risks influence theft, we asked the respondents, "How likely do you think it is that you would get caught, *if* you stole something that belonged to a patient?" The results are not encouraging. Less than half (41.6 percent) thought it would be "very likely" that they would get caught if they stole something. A nearly equal percentage (39.6 percent) actually thought it would be "very" or "somewhat unlikely" that they would get caught, and about 20 percent thought that getting caught would be only "somewhat likely."

We also asked employees to tell us what they thought would happen to them if they were caught stealing. As with the results on the perceived risk of getting caught, these results are not reassuring. The vast majority (98.7 percent) thought that something would happen, and the most likely result was termination of employment. More than 85 percent of the respondents indicated that they thought they would be fired if they were caught stealing. However, considerably less than half of the respondents, only 42.4 percent, thought they would be reported to the police. Thus, most nursing home employees apparently do not believe that if they are caught stealing from patients they will be subject to any sort of official legal sanction. At worst, they expect to lose their jobs. The failure of some nursing homes to report cases of theft or suspected theft by employees to the police is a serious flaw. It means that background checks on employees prior to hiring may not be very effective in screening out potential employees who may victimize the elderly. Although losing a job can be a significant hardship and in some cases a severe punishment for crime for some people, it might not be so bad for nursing home employees. Given the high employee turnover rate in many nursing homes, fired employees may not have too much difficulty finding employment in other homes.

Observations of Theft

Another way of uncovering information about theft in nursing homes is to ask employees to report whether they have observed or suspected other employees of stealing from patients. A total of 58 (5.7 percent) respondents reported observing their co-workers stealing from patients, and 194 (19.4 percent) suspected other employees of stealing. Three respondents said that they had both seen and suspected other employees of taking the possessions of patients. Taken together, a total of 255 respondents (25.5 percent of those answering this question) either saw or suspected other employees of stealing from patients.

That one-quarter of our respondents think that other employees are stealing from patients is sobering, but this result must be interpreted cautiously. It is possible, of course, that some respondents are mistaken in their suspicions about other employees. Thus, the percentage that reported only suspecting other employees of stealing might not reflect the actual amount of theft in a home. Indeed, we cannot determine whether respondents located in the same home are reporting on the same or different people. It is possible that a home may have only a small number of employees who are thieves, but their activities may be known to a large proportion of others. Thus, we cannot use this measure as an indicator of the proportion of employees involved in theft. Nevertheless, it indicates that a notable proportion of nursing home employees believe that employee theft occurs in their facilities.

We asked those who saw or suspected a fellow employee of theft what they had done about it. A majority (59.2 percent) said that they had reported the matter to their supervisor, but a sizeable minority did nothing. When asked how their supervisors handled their reports, the respondents gave a variety of answers. In 12.7 percent of the cases apparently "nothing happened to the employee," and in 37.6 percent of the cases, the respondents did not know or were not sure what happened to the employee. It is possible that in some of these cases, the employees' superiors determined that the suspicions of theft were not well-founded and hence no action was taken. In cases in which action was taken, the employees apparently were fired 12.7 percent of the time. Reprimands were administered in 11.3 percent of the cases, 10.7 percent were reported to the police, and 10.7 percent were "written up."

What Gets Stolen

When we asked those who admitted taking items from patients what they had taken, most of them would admit only to taking "food, candy, or flowers." Very few admitted taking money, jewelry, or other valuable personal possessions. Thus, from the perspective of those who admit taking items from patients, it appears that the thefts were perhaps not very significant, and that patients did not really lose personal possessions of much value. However, when we asked the same question of employees who said they had seen or suspected other employees of stealing, a different picture emerged. More than half (55.5 percent) said that they had seen or suspected other employees of taking "money, credit cards, or checks." Somewhat fewer (42.7 percent) thought that other employees were taking jewelry. Table 4.5 shows the frequency with which employees saw or suspected other employees of stealing certain items.

CONCLUSIONS ABOUT EMPLOYEES

As far as we can determine, the results presented in this chapter represent the first large-scale national data on theft from patients in nursing homes. Although our study is an advance over anecdotal reports on theft in nursing homes, it has limitations, which we have tried to point out in this chapter. The biggest shortcomings are the low overall response rate and the problem of respondent veracity on the

TABLE 4.5. What Gets Stolen: Employees' Observations and Suspicions of Items Stolen by Other Employees

Item	Percent reporting they saw or suspected other employees of stealing
Money, credit cards, checks	55.5
TVs, VCRs, radios	12.4
Jewelry	42.7
Clothing	32.1
Stamps	5.1
Food, candy, flowers	55.3
Knickknacks	18.6
Cosmetics, toiletries	19.7
Cigarettes, other tobacco products	17.9

theft items. Despite these limitations, several of our results are eye-opening.

Other researchers have found that nursing home employees whom patients abuse and who hold negative attitudes toward patients are more likely to engage in physical and psychological abuse of patients (Pillemer and Bachman-Prehn, 1991). We found a similar dynamic with respect to theft. Thieves reported significantly more abuse from patients and held more negative attitudes toward them than did non-thieves. The similarity between our findings on theft and the findings on physical abuse suggest that common causes may underlie different forms of abuse of patients. Employees may be motivated to behave aggressively toward patients because of their negative experiences with them. Aggression toward patients may be expressed directly by physically or psychologically assaulting patients or indirectly by stealing their belongings, or both. Even though the rate of self-reported theft was low, it is important to keep in mind that one-quarter of the respondents had reason to believe that their fellow employees were stealing from patients. Employees are in the rooms and around other employees and patients constantly. They are in the best position to be aware of what other employees are doing.

As far as we know, in the anonymous survey format used here, employees should have no reason to falsely report about their observations and suspicions of theft. Thus, we think it is particularly sobering that so many feel that thieves are relatively common in nursing homes. It is also sobering that employees apparently have relatively little to fear if they do steal. Many think that getting caught is not very likely, and most think that the worst that will happen to them is termination.

In addition to motivation, opportunity plays an important role in nursing home theft. Theft is related to occupational position, with those having the greatest access to patients—nursing aides—being most likely to self-report theft. As frontline caregivers, aides are responsible for 80 to 90 percent of direct patient care. They have near-unlimited access to patients' rooms, giving them frequent and intense contact with patients and their possessions. According to the routine activities perspective, this puts aides in close proximity to suitable targets under conditions of low to nonexistent protection and makes theft quite easy.

We do not wish to suggest that nursing aides should be blamed for all theft in nursing homes. Employees in other positions are dishonest as well. Furthermore, if our self-report results can be believed, the vast majority of aides do not steal from patients. Nevertheless, the low pay and stress combined with aides' relatively unmonitored access to patients' rooms and possessions creates conditions in which motivation and opportunity may all too often converge. Theft undoubtedly is the occasional by-product. The convergence of motivation and opportunity may be a structural feature of the organization of work in nursing homes that is difficult to eliminate.

Finally, our results have some policy implications. Recently, in recognition of problems in nursing homes, politicians and other policy-makers have called for stricter controls on hiring practices in the industry. Police background checks are mandatory in many states, and some have called for a national registry for employees who are dismissed from nursing homes for abusing patients (*Provider,* 1997). Such steps represent highly laudable efforts to protect patients, especially in the case of employees who have committed violent or sexual crimes against patients. However, their potential effectiveness against the problem of employee thieves is questionable. The effectiveness of police background checks, for example, depends on what is reported to the police and on how the police respond. Yet, our results suggest that in many nursing homes, employees who are suspected or even caught stealing from patients are more likely to be dismissed than reported to the police. Recall that more than half of our respondents thought that they would not be reported to the police if they were caught stealing.

The nursing home industry is not unique in the way it responds to employee misconduct. Other types of organizations seldom use criminal prosecution as punishment for theft (Hollinger and Clark, 1983). Job loss is, no doubt, a potent threat, but it may not be as severe a punishment as one would think. Getting another job as a nursing aide is probably not difficult in an industry for which the annual turnover rate for aides is estimated to be between 40 and 75 percent (Foner, 1994). Thus, although calls for police background checks represent a step in the right direction, more needs to be done to ensure that nursing homes report thefts to the police.

Chapter 5

The Victims and Their Families

Although the problem of theft from patients is widely recognized in the nursing home industry, insiders often blame this problem on the patients themselves rather than employees. It is not uncommon to hear nursing home administrators say that what really happens in most so-called "thefts" is that the object has simply been lost or misplaced by patients themselves, or administrators may claim that if a theft *has* occurred, other patients are responsible. Because many patients suffer from cognitive deficiencies, they make ideal scapegoats.

Despite the popularity of the self-report methodology, it suffers from the understandable shortcoming that offenders may not tell the truth about their activities. Hence, criminologists looking for other sources of information about crime have used another technique—the victimization survey. Victimization surveys are similar to **self-report surveys** in that they ask ordinary people about their experiences with crime. Since the mid-1960s, victimization surveys have become a mainstay of research on victims. The most well-known and important victimization survey is the National Crime Victimization Survey (NCVS), which is conducted annually (U.S. Department of Justice, 1998). The NCVS has revealed a wealth of information about the extent, distribution, and patterning of criminal victimization in the United States. Unfortunately, however, nursing home patients are not included in the sampling frame of the NCVS, so it can tell us nothing about their experiences. Thus, to supplement what we learned about theft from employees, we decided to conduct a victimization survey in our sample of nursing homes.

Although victimization surveys can provide much useful information about criminal events, it is difficult to use this approach in nursing homes. All surveys require that the respondent be able to read (in the case of self-administered instruments) and understand the survey questions and directions. Unfortunately, many nursing home residents suffer from cognitive deficiencies and are incapable of completing self-administered survey instruments.

In this situation, one option would be to administer surveys only to patients who are mentally capable of filling them out. We rejected this option for two reasons. First, ascertaining the mental capabilities of patients can be a complicated and time-consuming undertaking, which requires direct access to patients. We did not have the time or resources to conduct these evaluations. Another reason for not surveying only mentally competent patients is that patients who are not always mentally competent may be the most vulnerable victims for thieves. Because of their disabilities, they are unable to protect themselves and their property. They may even be unable to ask others for help or to report any losses that they do suffer. Hence, a victimization survey of only part of the patient population might grossly underestimate the true amount of victimization in nursing homes.

Nevertheless, it is important to try to get the victim's perspective on theft in nursing homes. Thus, we decided to ask family members of patients to serve as proxy respondents for their loved ones. We assumed that family members have sufficient awareness of the possessions that patients have and will notice if items are missing. In addition, we assumed that patients themselves might be more likely to report theft to their family members than to nursing home personnel.

Accordingly, we designed a questionnaire for family members that asked them to report on the experiences of their loved ones. Ideally, we would have liked to mail the family questionnaire to the families of all the patients in the nursing homes in our sample. However, most of the nursing homes in the sample did not feel at liberty to provide us with the names and addresses of family members. They were concerned that doing so might violate the family members' privacy. Hence, to distribute the family questionnaires, we provided each home with a display box for questionnaire packets and a large sign that invited family members to participate in the study. We asked the nursing home administrators to place the box in a conspicuous location in the home (for example, near the main entranceway in the lobby of the home) and use whatever means they could to encourage families to participate in the study. The family packets contained a copy of the questionnaire, another cover letter, and a business-return envelope. A total of 417 surveys were completed and returned to us. (For more details on the victimization survey, see the Appendix.)

FAMILY MEMBERS' REPORTS OF THEFT

In most cases it is impossible to determine with legal certainty exactly who, if anyone, is responsible when an item disappears from a patient's room. Within the industry, items that disappear usually are explained away as simply having been lost, misplaced, or taken by other patients. To take account of these alternative explanations of theft, we developed a series of questions regarding the disappearance of items. We began by asking family members whether, in the past year, they had noticed any of their relative's possessions missing. If they answered yes, then we asked a series of questions about how many times they had noticed items missing and what they thought had happened. Thus, we asked if they suspected that the missing items were "lost or misplaced by the nursing home," and if so, how many times this had happened. We asked the same questions in cases where they suspected the items were "inadvertently taken by other patients," "deliberately taken by other patients," or "deliberately stolen by someone who was not an employee or patient," or "deliberately stolen by a nursing home employee." Family members could report multiple instances of items missing and could give different reasons for the disappearances. For example, a respondent could report that she had noticed two items missing in the past year, and she thought that one item had simply been lost while the other item had been stolen by an employee. By giving respondents the opportunity to choose other non-theft scenarios, we hoped to arrive at a conservative estimate of the rate of victimization in nursing homes.

A total of 196 family members reported that they had noticed items missing in the past year. This number represents slightly less than half (47 percent) of the 417 family members in the sample. In seventy-nine cases, the family members thought that an employee had stolen the item. This represents 18.9 percent of the total sample, and 56 percent of those who reported missing items (see Table 5.1). As shown in Table 5.1, in the largest number of cases, family members reported that they thought the item had simply been lost or misplaced.

TABLE 5.1. Family Members' Beliefs About Missing Items

Explanation for missing item	Number	Percent of total sample[a]
Lost or misplaced	129	30.9
Inadvertently taken by other patient	65	15.6
Stolen by other patient	21	5.0
Stolen by someone else	16	3.8
Stolen by an employee	79	18.9

[a] Respondents may report on multiple instances.

Most of those who suspected theft by employees suspected that it had happened more than once in the past year. Thus, the family survey suggests that, in a year's span, close to one out of five nursing home patients is a victim of theft.

We cannot be certain about the accuracy of family members' suspicions of theft. However, because family members were more likely to say that missing items were simply lost or misplaced as opposed to being stolen, it suggests that they do not make accusations of theft lightly. If the suspicions of family members are reasonably accurate, the annual victimization rate for theft from patients in nursing homes is approximately one out of five. This victimization rate exceeds the rates at which elderly individuals living in the general community are victimized by personal theft and household crimes. According to the Bureau of Justice Statistics, in 1992 the rate of personal theft victimization for persons sixty-five and older was 16.3 per 1,000 (Whitaker, 1987). Between 1980 and 1985, the average victimization rate for household crimes (burglary, household larceny, and auto theft) for persons sixty-five and older was 102.7 per 1,000 (Whitaker, 1987). Although it is impossible to determine precisely, the victimization rate of 20 percent found in our survey may not be highly inflated. Indeed, because our sample of family members is heavily weighted toward families who visit often and who presumably care strongly about their relatives, it is possible that we have underestimated the victimization rate. Family members who visit frequently can report problems to the nursing home administration and advocate for their relatives, thereby providing a small amount of protection. Patients who are not visited regularly by family members may be more vulnerable to theft, because thieves may know that little chance exists that anyone will notice or complain about missing items. Thus, these patients may be more vulnerable to theft and have higher rates of victimization.

WHAT IS STOLEN?

If the items that patients and family members reported stolen were just little knickknacks, candy, or other small and trivial items, we might assume that perhaps they were not taken by employees. However, according to the family members who responded to our survey, most of the items that they reported stolen were not trivial. The item most frequently mentioned as stolen was clothing. Of the seventy-nine family members who reported thefts, 49 (or 62 percent) identified clothing. Our interviews confirmed this trend. According to one patient's niece in a nursing home that we visited:

> Theft continues to happen. Unfortunately, it's the staff that does it. My aunt had three new outfits among other things that I bought her for Christmas. Two months ago we looked for the beige outfit—gone. The tags had never been taken off. A brand-new crepe blouse—gone. She never put it on her back. It's the good stuff that gets taken. That's not including all the stuff she came with. I would say that at least 25 percent of her belongings are gone since she's been here.

The next most popular item to steal from patients was "money, credit cards, or checks," which was mentioned by twenty-seven (34.2 percent) of the respondents. These two items were followed, in order, by "cosmetics and toiletries" (24.4 percent), "food, candy, or flowers" (21.8 percent), "jewelry" (16.7 percent), "knickknacks" (10.3 percent), "TV, VCR, or radio" (8.9 percent), and "stamps" (1.3 percent).

We also asked family members to estimate the dollar value of stolen items. The response categories were "less than $5," "$5 to $10," "$10 to $50," and "more than $50." Their answers provide further evidence that the items taken from patients are not trivial. Of the seventy-four respondents who answered this question, only eleven, or 14.9 percent, said that the items stolen were worth $10 or less. More than three times as many (thirty-four) said the item was worth between $10 and $50, and almost as many (twenty-nine) said that it was worth more than $50. Thus, in almost 90 percent of the reported thefts the item or items was worth more than $10.

That clothing and money are the most frequently stolen items suggests that whoever took the items was acting rationally and with deliberation. A confused or mentally incompetent fellow patient would probably not pick up these types of items after wandering into another patient's room. From the perspective of opportunity theory, clothing is a particularly attractive target for rational predatory thieves, because it is readily available in patients' rooms, relatively easily concealed, and has immediate use or exchange value on the street. Unlike money or jewelry, which can be kept in lockboxes or safes, clothing usually is kept in closets or unlocked dressers where employees can easily gain access to it. The nature of the items reported stolen by family members argues against the claims of many in the nursing home industry that mentally incompetent patients are responsible for most theft in nursing homes. According to one nursing home worker:

> The employees know which patients to steal clothing from. They know which patients have good clothes and they routinely go to these patients' rooms to steal what was brought for them. Only the newest clothing would be missing, while the older, frayed items remained in the closet.

Who Is Victimized by Theft?

Outside of nursing homes, the risk of victimization for ordinary street crime is not spread evenly throughout the population. Some groups and types of individuals are at a much higher risk than others. Adolescents and young adults, for example, are at a much higher risk of victimization for most street crimes than are the middle-aged or elderly, and men are more likely to be victims of violent crime than women (Kamen, 2000; U.S. Department of Justice, 1998). Because so little information is available on the victims of theft in nursing homes, it is not known whether the factors that determine victimization risks in the general public also operate among nursing home populations. They may not. Nursing home populations are unique. They are more homogeneous regarding age than the general population, and the sex ratio of females to males is far higher in nursing homes than in the general population. Hence, it is likely that risk of victimization from theft in a nursing home may depend on different factors than it does in the general public.

To begin to explore this issue, we examined the relationship between standard demographic variables (sex, race, age, and marital status) and victimization by theft. We found little evidence that demographic characteristics significantly influence victimization. Virtually no difference in age between victims and non-victims existed. Likewise, no differences between whites and African Americans or between patients who were married versus those who were not married were found. The only notable pattern involved sex. Females were slightly more likely to be victimized than males (20.1 percent versus 15.5 percent, respectively), but the difference was not statistically significant.

Having established that demographic characteristics are unrelated to the likelihood of victimization by theft, we then explored whether other patient characteristics might be more important. We speculated that how long a patient has been in the nursing home, how often their family members visit, and the patient's level of awareness would be related to theft. Length of stay in the nursing home was significantly related to theft. For patients who had been in the nursing home for less than one year the victimization rate was approximately 10 percent, but it was more than twice as high for those who had been in the home for more than one year.

We had thought that the frequency of visits by family members would be related to theft, but we were unsure whether family visits would have a positive or a negative effect. On one hand, family visits might deter theft—if they increased guardianship—leading to a negative relationship between the frequency of visits and theft. On the other hand, family members who visit often may be more likely to notice things that are missing, leading to a positive relationship between visits and theft. The results suggested only slight evidence for a deterrence effect. Among family members who reported that they visited at least once every two weeks, the rate of theft was 18 percent compared to a slightly higher rate (23 percent) for those who visited less often. Thus, it is not clear that the frequency of family visits deters theft from patients.

Patients can act as their own guardians if they are aware of their surroundings and can monitor or secure their possessions. Hence, we thought that the level of the patient's awareness as reported by family members would be related to theft. This was not the case. We found virtually no difference in victimization rates between patients who were reported as being mentally aware most or all of the time and those who were aware only some of the time or rarely. The lack of a relationship between patient awareness and levels of theft may indicate that because of the way nursing homes are organized, patients can do little to protect themselves from predatory staff members. It appears that the more time a patient spends in a home, the more likely he or she is to lose something to theft.

Which Nursing Homes Are the Safest?

Nursing homes vary considerably in size. They range from small units that have fewer than fifty beds to large, mammoth structures with hundreds of patients. Nursing homes also vary in whether they are operated for profit or not. Both of these characteristics of homes may influence theft rates. For example, it is possible that because they are concerned with making money for-profit homes have poorer working conditions than not-for-profit homes. On the other hand, working conditions may actually be worse in nonprofit homes if they are poorly funded. Regardless of which type of home is a better place at which to work, poor pay or working conditions may be motives for theft from patients.

The size of a home may also influence opportunities for theft. For example, criminologists for some time have known that rates of street crime are higher in large urban settings than in small towns. One reason for the difference is that in large cities people do not know their neighbors as well as they do in small towns. It is more difficult for residents to recognize outsiders and to tell who belongs and who does not. These features of urban life are thought to reduce levels of informal social control in urban neighborhoods and to lead to increased crime rates (Sampson, 1987).

The same mechanisms may also apply in organizational settings. As organizations grow larger, it becomes less likely that all members of the organization will know one another personally; this may reduce the level of informal social control in the organization. Based on this reasoning we would expect theft rates to be higher in large nursing homes. We found some evidence in support of the idea that the characteristics of size and profit status in nursing homes influence theft rates. The following shows the victimization rates as reported by family members in small, medium, and large homes.

Small	12.7%
Medium	19.7%
Large	21.4%

Small homes have less than fifty beds, medium-sized homes have fifty to 199, and large-sized homes have more than 200 beds. There seems to be a clear relationship between size and rate of theft. In small homes, only 12.7 percent of the family members reported suspecting that items had been stolen from their relatives, but in large homes the rate was 21.4 percent. However, no relationship between profit status and theft was apparent. The victimization rate in for-profit homes was 19.1 percent, compared to 17.9 percent in not-for-profit homes.

To explore whether the combination of size and profit status influences theft more strongly than either one of these characteristics individually, we grouped homes into six categories based on size and profit status. Then, we investigated reported theft rates in the categories. The results suggest that the large nonprofit homes have the highest theft rates, while small nonprofit homes have the lowest rates (see Table 5.2). Of the twenty-one family members whose relatives were patients in a large nonprofit home, six, or 28.6 percent, reported theft, but of the twenty-two family members whose relatives were in small

TABLE 5.2. Victimization Rate by Size and Type of Home

Size of home	For profit	Not for profit
Small	19.6% (51)	0.0% (22)
Medium	19.4% (206)	19.6% (51)
Large	19.0% (63)	28.6% (21)

nonprofit homes, none reported theft. Theft rates were virtually identical at around 19 percent for all other types of homes. These results are suggestive, but they must be interpreted with caution because they are not statistically significant and are based on small sample sizes. It is possible that if we had larger, more representative samples of individuals in the different types of homes, we would not find such notable differences in theft rates.

What Happens Afterward

After a theft has come to light, victims can respond in a variety of ways. They may do nothing or they may report the incident to the nursing home. It is well-known that more than half of all street crimes are not reported to the police (U.S. Department of Justice, 1998). Victims fail to report crimes for a variety of reasons, such as fear of retaliation or belief that the police can do little to help. Similar reasons may prevent the victims of theft in nursing homes from reporting the incident to the nursing home. We asked the respondents who indicated that they suspected theft by employees whether they reported the incident to the nursing home and, if they did, what happened as a result of their report. Close to two-thirds (62.8 percent) said that they did report the missing item to the nursing home. The remainder did not report or were not sure whether anyone else had reported the theft. In the vast majority of cases, reporting to the home did not lead to salutary results. Items were recovered in only 13 percent of the cases, and no one reported that the thief or thieves were caught. Probably because no one was ever identified as the thief, none of the suspected thefts were reported to the police by the nursing homes. Not surprisingly, only 16 percent of the respondents said they were satisfied with the way the nursing home responded to the incident.

Theft in a Nursing Home

The fact that theft is prevalent increases the residents' knowledge of their insecurity and ability to control their environment. Everything is stealable. . . . Much of the social worker's time is spent answering phone calls from relatives who are angry that their parents underwear or new clothing that they bought cannot be located. (Shield, 1988, p. 159)

CONCLUSION

In this chapter, we have reported results of one of the first victimization surveys in nursing homes focusing on theft. Although the findings must be interpreted with caution, at a minimum they indicate that nursing home patients often lose their possessions and that, at least as far as their family members are concerned, a notable proportion of these losses are the result of theft by staff members. As we have noted at several points in this chapter, for the cases discussed here, it is impossible to prove that the missing items were indeed stolen. But in light of the apparent reluctance of family members to make the accusation of theft lightly and considering the nature of the items most frequently stolen, we think it is reasonable to conclude that employee theft from patients is not uncommon. Indeed, for the elderly the risk of theft victimization may be higher inside than it is outside of nursing homes.

Chapter 6

Preventing and Reducing Theft

> An 86-year-old nursing home patient awoke [and] . . . discovered that during the night her finger had been stripped of life's last two mementos: the diamond ring inherited from her father and the engagement ring that her husband had slipped on her finger during a romantic canoe ride. (Rogers, 1996, p. 1)

Theft continues to be one of the most prevalent problems in nursing homes. Yet, so few official complaints are filed in relation to the number of actual incidents it seems that it has become an accepted and expected occurrence in nursing homes. According to the **American Association of Retired Persons** (1998), the best protection against theft is not to bring anything valuable into the nursing home. However, even items that are not valuable are stolen!

Drawing on insights from the routine activities theory, Clarke (1995) developed the **situational theory,** which is a crime prevention approach that focuses on reducing the opportunity for certain types of crime to occur by increasing the risks and difficulties associated with committing them. Crime reduction, according to Clarke, can be achieved by managing and manipulating the environment. His practical and commonsense approach includes a set of opportunity-reducing strategies that can be adapted for patients as well as nursing homes. They are listed in the following section.

THEFT PRECAUTIONS FOR PATIENTS

Target Hardening

- One of the most common ways to protect property in patients' rooms is to put locks on drawers, especially bedside tables, and on closet doors. Only the patient or his or her representative and the administrator should have a key. If the patient has a small refrigerator in his or her room, it also should be secured with a lock to prevent the theft of its contents.

- The **Senior Crimestoppers** program provides lockboxes for each patient in a participating facility. These boxes are mounted in the patients' rooms so that they can secure some of their possessions.
- Televisions, VCRs, radios, and other large valuables belonging to the patients should be fastened down to make them difficult to remove.
- Patients should wear ring guards or have their rings downsized to make it more difficult to have them slipped off their fingers.
- They should never leave money and jewelry out in the open, as it only creates opportunities for thieves.
- Patients may want to use a change purse to carry small amounts of money during the day and can pin it to their clothing for safekeeping.

Target Removal

- A majority of nursing homes rely on a safe in the facility's office to protect patients' money and other valuables. The drawback of the facility safe is that it does not allow the patients easy access to their belongings.
- Fake rings and other jewelry may be given to the patients to wear while the genuine articles are kept at home by their families.

Identify Property

- An inventory should be made of the patients' possessions at the time of admittance and periodically updated.
- Patients' clothing should be marked with indelible pens, monograms, or name tags that are ironed on or sewed into all garments. One daughter used a black marking pen to write the name of her wheelchair-bound mother in large letters on the back of all her clothes.

- Some families take home all their relatives' clothing to launder, because nursing homes often blame the loss of garments on laundry mix-ups and difficulty in reading the patients' names.
- Mark property such as television sets, VCRs, and radios with an engraving pencil.
- Have pictures made of the patients' valuable items. These are helpful for documentation as well as identification.

THEFT PRECAUTIONS FOR NURSING HOMES

Access Control

- Limit access to the home as much as possible by restricting the number of entrances and exits.
- Some nursing homes use a sign-in and sign-out book for visitors and provide them with badges.

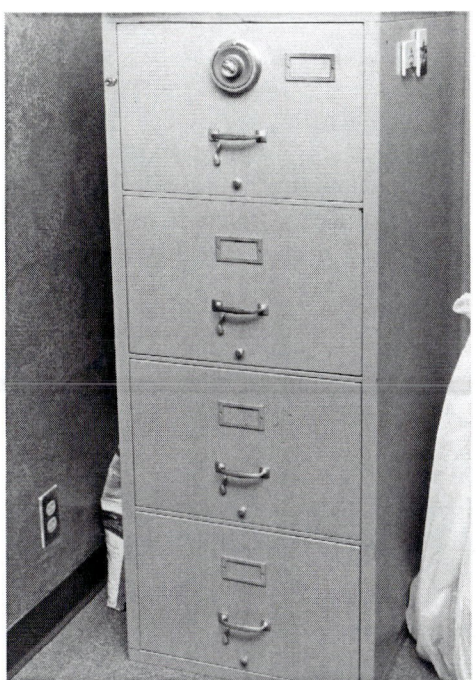

A safe in a nursing home.

Exit Screening

- Use clear trash bags to help prevent employees from taking home patients' belongings.
- Have female employees carry clear plastic purses so that the contents of their purses can be monitored when they leave.

Formal Surveillance

- Install a burglar alarm system as well as a camera at unsupervised doors.
- Use closed-circuit televisions to provide surveillance in the halls and stairwells. The use of cameras with small lenses in patients' rooms has been the subject of nationwide debates. It has been argued that these cameras could zoom in on a bedside table drawer, closet, or other places where valuables are kept without invading the patient's privacy. In addition to protecting the patients against theft, these cameras (nicknamed "granny cams") also have the potential to reduce incidents of abuse. Opponents of this proposal, including nursing home administrators and workers, argue that the presence of these cameras will invade the privacy of patients. They fear that cameras would create an atmosphere of distrust, increase employee stress, and make nursing homes undesirable places to work.
- Have a crime prevention officer from the local police department conduct a building security survey and occasionally visit the facility.

Surveillance by Employees

- Alert employees to report any unusual occurrences. Have an in-house hotline for employees to report these occurrences as well as witnessing theft from a patient. The Senior Crimestoppers program offers round-the-clock access to a tip hotline. All callers are guaranteed anonymity. Rewards of up to $1,000 are offered for information that helps bring situations to a successful conclusion.
- Have employees work in pairs if staffing permits so that they are not alone in a patient's room at any time and can "keep an eye" on one another. Also, if possible, have employees leave in groups at the end of their shifts to help provide peer surveillance.

Present Protection

To prevent the theft of presents prior to Christmas, some nursing homes take the packages as patients receive them, put their names on them, and lock them in a special closet. The packages are then distributed on Christmas morning.

REPORTING OF THEFT

To paraphrase an old maxim: "He who hesitates reporting a theft has less chance of recovering the loss." In one instance a woman came back to her room after a meal and saw an aide going through her dresser drawers and taking out her diamond engagement ring. The woman did not know what to do. She finally called her son the next day and told him what happened. The following day he reported the theft to the police. By then, the ring and the aide were long gone.

The sooner a theft is reported and investigated, the better the chance of getting the stolen item returned. But some patients and their families do not even bother reporting a theft. One reason is that they think the home is not concerned about their loss and will take no action. Another reason is that, because of the close contact patients have with many of the thieves, they are fearful of being threatened or suffering retaliation from them. Finally, some patients are afraid no one will believe them when they say something has been stolen. In one case a woman whose watch was taken reported that she saw the aide slip the watch off her arm. No one believed her. Luckily, the aide was foolish enough to wear the watch to work. She was immediately fired.

Patients and their families should be encouraged to report a theft immediately and fill out a missing-property report form. The form should be simple to use and the reporting process easy to understand. In some cases of theft, the police should be notified by the family or the home.

Each report of theft must be promptly followed up and investigated by the administration. Otherwise, dishonest employees think that the administrators do not care. Prompt investigation of every case of suspected theft sends the message that theft is taken seriously by the home and will not be tolerated.

THEFT PREVENTION TRAINING PROGRAMS

Although stealing from nursing home patients is an old problem, the idea of a specialized training program to prevent or reduce its occurrence is a relatively new approach. Such a program should help the employees

- Understand the sentimental value and important memories that many of the patients' belongings hold for them. Some of these items are irreplaceable—at least in the minds of their owners.
- Know that even though some cognitively impaired patients cannot appreciate or are not aware of their possessions, stealing from them will not be tolerated.
- Provide knowledge about how to deal with troublesome or demented patients. Some employees misinterpret their aggressive behavior and retaliate by stealing from them. (See Chapter 9 for programs designed to prevent abuse.)

Talking freely about theft helps remove the veil of secrecy surrounding it. A theft prevention program should involve not only the staff, but the patients and families as well. Winning the support and cooperation of both groups is essential for a successful program. Make them partners in theft prevention and ask them for suggestions in dealing with it. In addition, employees should be made aware of the issue of theft; sometimes they can help solve this problem.

The program should also stress the importance of being aware of what is happening in the home. Any behavior that seems out of the ordinary or suspicious should be reported. The following case illustrates this point:

Frances had received some money from her family for her birthday. A nurse passed by the room the next day and saw an aide in there that was not normally there. She said that she did not think much of it, as she was busy and did not have time to stop. Later, another patient claimed money had been stolen from him. The administrator began to look for the missing money. When they questioned Frances, she noticed that the money given to her for her birthday was also missing. The nurse remembered the aide he had seen in Frances's room earlier. After questioning the aide, the administrator discovered that she was responsible for both thefts.

Finally, an essential part of a theft program is to stop stealing before it starts. Carefully screening prospective employees (we discuss screening in Chapter 9) and warning new employees about the consequences they will face if they steal from patients are two important steps in this direction.

PART III:
PHYSICAL AND MENTAL MALTREATMENT

Chapter 7

Physical Abuse and Neglect

The abuse of the elderly is not a recent phenomena; it dates back to other places and other eras.

> Elder abuse represents an unbroken saga in the relations between adults and their elders. These cultural products give testimony to persistent intergenerational cruelty. This tradition of abuse however is challenged by the equally forceful norm of respect for elders. Thus respect and disdain together define intergenerational relations. (Reinharz, 1986, p. 25)

In many precivilized societies, death was the solution when an elderly person became a burden to his or her family or community. In some societies, death occurred indirectly either through abandonment, segregation, or neglect. In other places, death was required by a definite cultural prescription; the elderly were killed outright or committed suicide.

ABANDONMENT, SEGREGATION, AND NEGLECT

In the past, it was not uncommon for many groups to abandon their elderly when moving from place to place or changing camps. In most cases, it was the only practical thing to do since strenuous travel for old and infirm persons was not feasible, and to carry sick, frail persons on a long journey was not possible. Generally, when the elderly were left behind, they were provided with shelter and a small amount of food and water.

In Australia, the Euahlayi would leave old and ailing persons behind with a young companion whose job it was to bury them when they died. Among the Creek Indians it was an approved custom to offer the elderly a choice between abandonment and voluntary death.

In some societies, when a person became old and incapacitated, he or she was segregated from the rest of the group. The Hottentots of South Africa, the Bushmen of South Africa, and the Hopi and Crow Indians placed their elderly in small huts with a few provisions and left them to die. Similarly, Eskimos were walled up in igloos until they froze to death or were set adrift on an ice floe. It is said that in ancient times in some remote Japanese villages when there was an extreme shortage of food, old people were carried up to the mountains and abandoned so that younger persons could survive. (See Figure 7.1.)

The elderly of the Yakut of Siberia were completely neglected by their families. They eventually died from lack of food and care. Sieroshevski (1896) describes their harsh treatment:

> I have seen living skeletons . . . who hid in corners, only emerging when there were not strangers there, to come nearer the fire. They let you perish slowly of cold and hunger in a corner, dying not like human beings but like brute beasts. . . . They begrudge you food, they drive you away from the fire, they begin to curse you for every trifle, they do not care for your illness, and so bedded in the corner, you die slowly from cold. (p. 227)

In some societies the outright killing of aged persons was regarded as the proper thing to do. When the Eskimos of the Hudson Bay area became old and dependent, the group strangled them by tying strings around their necks, and hoisted them to their deaths. Among the Banks Islanders and Melanesians, it was common for elderly infirm persons to beg their friends and families to bury them. The Samoans at one time believed that it was an honor and a tribute to be buried alive and many old people, especially those of high status, looked forward to such a death.

GOVERNMENT REFORM COMMITTEE

The study of the abuse of older people in our society may be traced back to the nursing home scandals of the late 1960s and 1970s (e.g.,

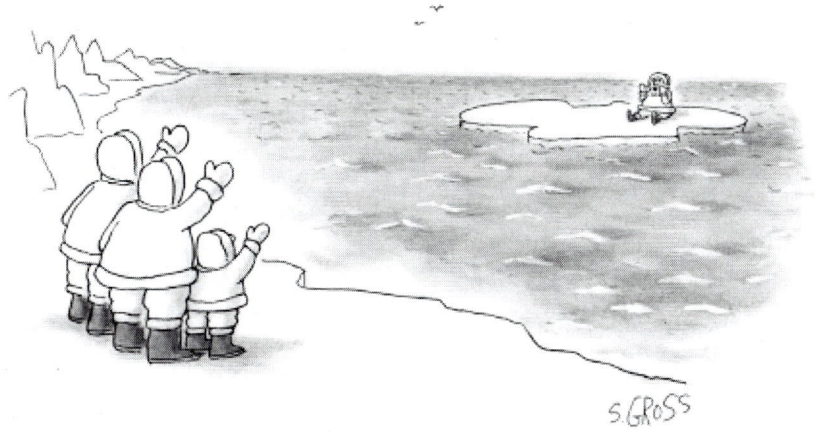

"Are you sure this ice floe is going to pass by the nursing home?"

FIGURE 7.1. Satirical Cartoon Regarding Treatment of the Elderly (© The New Yorker Collection 1999 Sam Gross from cartoonbank.com. All Rights Reserved.)

Stannard, 1973), which led to an examination of nursing home standards. This examination resulted in the passage of **nursing home reforms** contained in the Omnibus Budget Reconciliation Act of 1987. These reforms included such mandates as giving patients the right to be free from physical and mental abuse and corporal punishment.

Recently, a nationwide series of reports on the abuse of nursing home residents was prepared by the Minority Staff of the Special Investigations Division of the Committee on Government Reform for Members of Congress. These reports document instances during which nursing homes were cited for serious abuse violations. They are considered to be representative of nursing home abuse in the United States for the two-year period of January 1999 through January 2001 (Minority Staff of the House Committee on Government Reform, 2001).

These reports revealed that 30 percent, or 5,283, of the 17,000 nursing homes in the United States were cited for abuse violations during this period. All the violations had the potential to cause more than minimal harm to the patients, but 1,345 nursing homes were cited for an abuse violation that actually harmed patients. An additional 256 homes were cited for abuse violations that resulted in death or serious injury or placed patients in immediate jeopardy of death or serious injury (see Table 7.1).

It is likely that the findings in this report underestimate the incidence of abuse in nursing homes because researchers have reported that abuse cases are especially likely to go undetected and unreported. Law enforcement agencies generally do not treat crimes against the elderly in nursing homes in the same way they do other crimes. Yet, the percentage of homes cited for abuse violations during annual state inspections has almost tripled in four years. In 1996, it was 5.9 percent, and by 2000 it had reached 16 percent. Some of this increase is probably due in part to better enforcement efforts by state inspectors and improved reporting of abuse violations. In addition, in 1997 Congress repealed a provision of nursing home law known as the **"Boren Amendment."** This amendment guaranteed that nursing homes would receive "reasonable and adequate" Medicaid reimbursements to provide quality care. Since its repeal, Medicaid reimbursement rates have not kept pace with the rising costs of nursing home care. It has been argued that the lower Medicaid reimbursement rates have made it more difficult for nursing homes to recruit and retain quality staff, which has resulted in a higher rate of abuse violations (see Figure 7.2).

The state inspection reports and citations document that many patients were subjected to serious physical abuse by nursing staff. Physical abuse may be defined as any act that causes pain or injury. Such abuse ranges from bruises and broken bones, to lacerations and even

TABLE 7.1. Nursing Homes Cited for Abuse (1999-2000)

Abuse	Number of homes	Percent of homes
Potential for harm	3,682	21.3%
Actual harm to patients	1,345	7.8%
Serious injury or death	256	1.5%
Total	5,283	30.6%

Source: The Minority Staff of the House Committee on Government Reform, 2001.

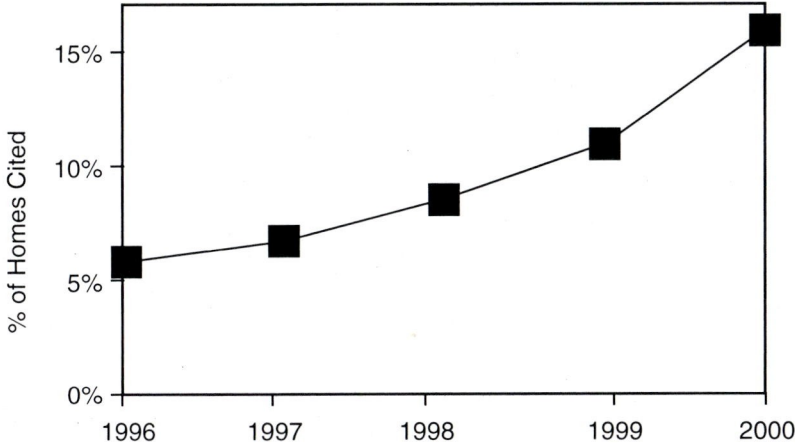

FIGURE 7.2. The Percentage of Nursing Homes Cited for Abuse Violations in Annual Inspections (1996-2000) (*Source:* The Minority Staff of the House Committee on Government Reform, 2001, p. 7).

death. For example, Marshall, seventy-eight, was suffering from **Alzheimer's disease**. He died in a nursing home not from disease, but from homicide:

> Ten days before his death two nursing aides saw an orderly coming out of Marshall's room. When they went in his room they discovered that Marshall had a cut on his lip and eyelid. Earlier that day, they heard the orderly threatening to hurt Marshall for spitting medicine on his shirt. According to the aides, the orderly enjoyed tormenting patients. Five days later Marshall was found with a badly cut lip and his gown was torn. He was taken to a hospital, stitched up and brought back. The next morning, Marshall was found slumped over in his wheelchair and rushed again to the hospital. He died four days later from a subdural hematoma—a collection of blood in the brain from being beaten. The orderly was sentenced to 15 years in prison for first-degree elder abuse. (Munz, 2004)*

---

*Reprinted with permission of the St. Louis Post-Dispatch, copyright 2004.

TYPES OF PHYSICAL ABUSE

Although only a small proportion of nursing home employees abuse patients, the presence of abusive staff can affect the quality of care and peace of mind of large numbers of nursing home patients (For public opinion on the occurrence of abuse, see Exhibit 7.1). The following are some indicators of physical abuse:

contusions or lesions	gag marks
eye injuries	sprains
pinch marks	bruises
welts	missing teeth
scratches	burns
fractures	puncture wounds
human bite marks	cuts
patches of hair missing and/or	choke marks
bleeding below the scalp	dislocation

Pillemer and Moore (1989) interviewed 577 nurses and nursing home aides by telephone to assess the nature and extent of patient abuse. They found that 36 percent of the sample said they had seen at least one incident of physical abuse in the past year and as many as 10 percent reported that they had committed one or more abusive acts. Pushing, grabbing, shoving, or pinching a patient were reported by 3 percent of the respondents, as was hitting or slapping a patient. The researchers identified factors such as low job satisfaction, treating the

---

EXHIBIT 7.1. Survey Question Addressed to the Public

Do you think the following is something that happens to almost all nursing home residents, many of them, some, or hardly any?

Residents are abused by the staff.

Almost all	Many	Some	Hardly any
5%	9%	53%	30%

Source: The NewsHour with Jim Lehrer/Kaiser Family Foundation/Harvard School of Public Health National Survey on Nursing Homes, September 2001.

patients like children, and high levels of conflict with patients as being related to abusive behavior. Other researchers have associated certain demographics with patient abuse. These include being male and younger, and having lower educational levels and less experience working in a home (e.g., Penner et al., 1984; Baltz and Turner, 1977).

Payne and Cikovic (1995) examined the abuse of nursing home patients by analyzing 488 cases throughout the nation, reported to the Medicaid Fraud Control Unit between 1987 and 1992. They found physical abuse to be the most frequent type of mistreatment. It occurred in 411 cases (84.2 percent). Acts of physical abuse included burning a patient with a cigarette, hitting a patient with an object, and repeatedly slapping a 104-year-old wheelchair-bound patient. Although all occupational groups were involved in abusive behavior, nursing aides comprised the largest group of abusers at nearly 62 percent. This is not surprising; they not only are the largest occupational group in nursing homes, but they also have more contact with patients than do other employees. When Harris and Benson (1999) surveyed forty-seven nursing homes by mailed questionnaires, they found 3.5 percent of *all* the employees in the nursing homes reported they had shoved or pinched a patient, while 3.4 percent reported hitting or slapping a patient.

Elder mistreatment may be divided into two types: **sadistic abusers** and **reactive abusers** (Ramsey-Klawsnik, 1995). The case at the beginning of the chapter regarding an elderly man who was repeatedly beaten by an orderly is an example of sadistic abuse. In another nursing home:

> A patient was attacked by an orderly who hit him in the eye. The patient said the orderly was in a "rage." The patient's roommate also complained about the rough treatment by the same person, stating, "He's sadistic. It seems he likes to hurt people." Upon review of the nursing home's personnel files, state inspectors found that he had been alleged to have sexually molested a female patient and had numerous disciplinary and work-related complaints. The sexual abuse allegation had not been investigated or reported to the state. (Minority Staff of the House Committee on Government Reform, 2001, p. 10)

A nursing aide who suddenly loses his or her self-control and chokes a patient in response to being hit with an object or having his or her hair pulled would be called a "reactive abuser." The major difference between the two types is intent. The sadistic abuser has malicious intent whereas the reactive abuser does not. The sadistic abuser's act is premeditated whereas the reactive abuser is spontaneous and unplanned (see Table 7.2). In fact, the reactive abuser initially may be well-intentioned, but may lash out in anger or impatience.

Restraints

There are two kinds of restraints: physical and chemical. Physical restraints, as the name implies, are devices attached to or adjacent to a patient's body that restrict range of motion. They cannot be easily removed by the patient. Physical restraints are used in nursing homes mainly to prevent falling, to protect treatment devices, and to control behavioral symptoms such as physical and verbal aggression and wandering. Restraints have been criticized because their use may lead to a number of health problems including decreased muscle tone, pressure ulcers, circulatory obstruction, and even death. Federal regulations require that they should be used only when other, less severe alternatives fail to meet a patient's needs and the benefits outweigh

TABLE 7.2. Types of Elder Abusers

Sadistic abuser	Reactive abuser
Have abusive or sadistic personalities and often criminal intent	Lack abusive, sadistic, or criminal intent
Purposely inflict pain and suffering; may enjoy terrifying their victims	Well-intentioned, competent caregivers; may lash out when overwhelmed by stress
Often lack guilt, shame, or remorse regarding the harm they have inflicted upon their victims	Often experience guilt and shame regarding their harmful actions
Often deny the allegations and may express outrage that they have been accused	Often acknowledge their abusive actions

Source: Adapted from Ramsey-Klawsnik (1995).

the potential risks. When restraints are used, patients should be carefully supervised. They also should be released and exercised every two hours to offset potential problems caused by immobility.

As a result of the Nursing Home Reform Law, popularly known as OBRA (1987), the number of nursing home patients who are physically restrained has declined dramatically. For example, in 1989, 40 percent of nursing home patients were physically restrained. Recently, the percentage has dropped to 10.5 percent (American Health Care Association, 2001). The following is one nursing home patient's view on restraints:

> Why take that dignity away from them, why take that independence away from them? It's going to come in time anyway soon enough. So sometimes we get a broken hip, and persons may end up in bed or a chair, but at least they had 40 years of walking versus 20 years of being tied in a chair. (O'Brien, 1989)

The decision of whether to use a physical restraint often creates a dilemma for the nursing staff. Is it better to risk having patients harm themselves or to use restraints, which may create other problems? For instance, a ninety-year-old woman fell when trying to climb over the side rails in her bed, and on another occasion when trying to get up from her wheelchair without assistance. Both times she was taken to the hospital with lacerations to her head from the falls. At this point, the nursing home decided restraints were needed to avoid additional injuries.

Some of the most common types of physical restraints are:

- A **gerichair** with an attached tray so that it cannot be easily removed. Sometimes a lap cushion is used instead of a tray.
- Alarms that sound when the patient gets up, but do not restrict a patient's range of motion.
- Waist or vest restraints; used to secure persons to chairs or beds.
- Bed rails, which are sometimes not considered to be restraints even though they help prevent the patient from getting up and falling out of bed.

Psychoactive drugs, often referred to as **"chemical restraints,"** are mind-altering drugs that are used to control behavioral symptoms that affect thinking, feeling, and reacting. They include tranquilizers, sedatives, and antidepressants. If used properly, they are helpful in controlling a number of behavioral and psychiatric problems. However, caution must be exercised in their use; they have the potential to cause a number of negative side effects, such as a drop in blood pressure, which can lead to falls, agitation, and being sleepy and unresponsive (Burger et al., 2000). For example, a daughter whose mother was in a nursing home noted:

> They had her on Haldol. We'd see her and she would be asleep. We would say, "Mother," and she wouldn't respond. I said they were giving her too much. I don't want to see her in that way. It wasn't doing her any good. It was easing their problem . . . getting her out of the way. We would go in there and she couldn't eat. She was just out of it. (AARP, 1998, p. 30)

Nursing homes too often use psychoactive drugs to control the behavior of aggressive or agitated patients. This might be done for the convenience of the facility, and ignores the problems of the patient. Although the nursing home reforms contained in OBRA 1987 mandated that nursing home patients should be free from unnecessary psychoactive drug use, especially when such medications are used only as chemical restraints, 50 percent of all nursing home patients were receiving them in 1999 and 2000 (American Health Care Association, 2001).

Another form of drug misuse in nursing homes exists: mistakes made by the nursing staff in dispensing and administering medications. Such mistakes include giving the wrong medications or incorrect dosages. Improper dispensing of drugs in nursing homes can cause serious consequences and even death. For example, an elderly man in a nursing home who was diabetic and had not eaten in two days was given a large dose of insulin. As a result, he lapsed into a coma and died.

SEXUAL ABUSE

The **sexual abuse** of women as well as men in nursing homes is perpetrated by their caregivers and others who have access to patients. Sexual abouse is defined as engaging in sexual contact with a person without his or her consent. It involves physically forcing or threatening a person to have sexual activity or engaging in sexual activity with a victim who is incapable of granting informed consent (Ramsey-Klawsnik, 1996). Sexual abuse ranges from fondling and inappropriate touching to rape. The following two cases illustrate how offenders often seek victims who are rendered helpless due to impairments.

> A 61-year-old stroke victim was raped repeatedly over a two-year period by a nursing home orderly who was found to have attacked ten other women in the home, nine of them Alzheimer's patients. Her pleas for help, according to a suit filed by her husband against the home, were dismissed as symptoms of dementia. (Foote, 1995, p. C1)

> A male . . . nurse was discovered just after midnight by a nursing aide having sex with a 74-year-old woman with Alzheimer's . . . [and] charged with one count of first-degree sexual abuse and sentenced to five years of probation. The case did not go to trial because the elderly woman was unable to testify. (Rowden, 2000 p. 3)

Elderly people with mental and physical disabilities are especially at risk because they are unable to seek help during or after an attack and they lack credibility even if the assault is reported. Teaster and colleagues (2000) found that the majority of cases of sexual abuse were not prosecuted because of insufficient evidence or because the elderly victims were not able to participate in the prosecution.

A study done by the U.S. General Accounting Office (2002) revealed that family members, staff, and management often delay reporting alleged abuse, as the following example illustrates:

A patient reported to a **licensed practical nurse** that she had been raped in the nursing home. Although the nurse recorded this information in the patient's chart, she did not notify the nursing home management. She also allegedly discouraged the resident from telling anyone else. Two months later, the resident was admitted to a hospital for unrelated reasons and told hospital officials that she had been raped. It was not until the hospital officials notified police of the patient's complaint that an investigation was conducted. Investigators then discovered that the patient had also informed her daughter of the incident, but the daughter, apparently not believing her mother, had dismissed it. The patient later told police that she did not report the incident to nursing home staff because she did not want to cause trouble. The case was closed because the patient could not describe the alleged perpetrator. However, the nurse was counseled about the need to immediately report such incidents.

NEGLECT

Neglect is possibly one of the most demeaning aspects of living in a nursing home. The patient who must depend on others to perform the most basic and personal tasks suffers from both the loss of self-esteem and control over his or her body. In this context, neglect refers to the refusal or failure of nursing home personnel to fulfill their caregiving obligations.

Neglect often occurs when aides are overworked or when homes are short staffed; often, this results in aides not having the time to deal with difficult patients. Neglect may be passive or active. **Active neglect** is the act of deliberately refusing to fulfill caregiving obligations (e.g., a caregiver who willfully withholds medicine from a patient). **Passive neglect** refers to nondeliberately failing to fulfill caregiving obligations (e.g., a nursing aide with a heavy workload who leaves incontinent patients unchanged for long periods of time). One daughter of a nursing home patient wrote:

> There have been times when I visited my mother and the smell that hits my face from her unchanged soiled Depends is beyond belief. I have been there when they changed her without washing her, and then they open the window in her room while she is there on a cold winter day. . . . It appears that this nursing home is trying to kill my mother, if not of pneumonia or uncleanness, perhaps by stripping her of all her dignity and independence. (National Citizen's Coalition for Nursing Home Reform, 2001b, p. 1)

According to an abuse investigator:

> Residents who are the most in need, the most disabled, [and] the most infirmed have a tendency to be neglected more than the residents who are able to speak for themselves and request help.

Also residents who have no family coming in or no regular visitors seem to be more prone to be neglected. (Shaw, 1998)

One of the most common problems associated with neglect is **decubitus ulcers,** commonly called **pressure sores** or bedsores. Bedsores are skin lesions resulting from unrelieved pressure, which causes damage to underlying tissue. They usually occur over bony parts of the body such as heels, hips, and the sacrum. If the pressure continues, the wound deepens and the bone underneath becomes visible. In one nursing home alone, state inspectors found more than sixty patients suffering from this condition (Minority Staff of the House Committee on Government Reform, 2001). At-risk patients require frequent repositioning or turning to keep pressure off the wound. This condition occurs more often in persons who are bedridden or wheelchair bound.

In one incident, a nursing home patient was sent to the hospital for the treatment of a bedsore. The hospital staff treated the condition and gave the nursing home instructions on how to keep the wound clean and dressed. Several days later, family members noticed an odor and seepage from the wound and asked that the patient be returned to the hospital. The hospital staff looked at the bandage and saw that it had not been changed as they instructed. When the bandage was removed, insects crawled and flew out of the wound (Malone, 2000).

A ninety-one-year-old woman in a nursing home developed a bedsore on her leg from negligent care. As time went on, the sore worsened. At the request of the patient's daughter, the woman was taken to see a specialist. The specialist said that the only thing he could suggest was to amputate the woman's leg. At her advanced age and considering her frail condition, the decision was made to let the bedsore take its course. Gangrene eventually set in, and the woman died.

This chapter identified and described the abused elderly patients and their abusers. Such inhumane conditions in nursing homes that result in serious harm as well as death for this frail segment of our population can no longer be tolerated.

Chapter 8

Psychological Abuse and Neglect

Remember the old childhood expression "Sticks and stones may break my bones but names will never hurt me"? Name-calling is only one of many kinds of psychological or emotional abuse found in nursing homes. Others include being humiliated, chastised, made fun of, yelled at, cursed, treated as a child, ignored, insulted, or threatened. Often, psychological abuse can hurt a patient just as much, and sometimes more, than physical abuse. Podnieks (1987) distinguishes between physical and psychological mistreatment by labeling the former *overt* (e.g., hitting and slapping) and the latter *covert* (e.g., cursing and threatening). Many times, physical abuse is also accompanied by psychological abuse or may eventually lead to it. Unlike physical abuse, psychological abuse leaves no visible scars, but its effects are reflected in the behavior of the victim. Such behavior may include fearfulness, downcast eyes, or withdrawal from others. Although psychological mistreatment leaves no outward wounds, nevertheless, as one writer noted, "it bruises the soul." Psychological abuse may be defined as the infliction of emotional pain or threat of injury resulting in mental distress. Examples include the use of demeaning language, ridiculing or yelling at the patient, as well as ignoring him or her. One daughter relates the following case of psychological abuse:

> One night I went to visit there was a sleet storm. . . . I had to spend the night in the empty bed in mother's room. The nursing assistants came in to change mother. First they scolded her, using obscene language, for wetting the bed. Then, they told her snakes were around her feet and she better move them. Mother is unable to move. (AARP, 1998, p. 31)

TYPES OF PSYCHOLOGICAL ABUSE

Pillemer and Moore's (1989) survey of nursing home aides and nurses revealed that 81 percent of the respondents had observed at least one psychologically abusive incident in the preceding year. The most frequent type of psychological abuse was yelling at patients, which was reported by 33 percent of the staff, followed by insulting or swearing at them (10 percent). Factors related to the staff's verbal abuse of patients were job dissatisfaction, a stressful personal life, high levels of job burnout, and conflict with patients. Furthermore, the researchers found that staff members who treated the patients like children were at greatest risk of engaging in psychologically abusive behavior.

The following are some indicators commonly seen among victims of psychological abuse:

anger	passivity
agitation	depression
nervousness, trembling	cowering
evasiveness	fearfulness
shame	withdrawal
unwillingness to communicate	disorientation
confusion	sudden behavioral changes

Infantilization

A common problem in many nursing homes is infantilizing patients and treating them as children instead of as mature adults. Kayser-Jones (1981) cites the following examples:

> One day a nursing aide walked into the lounge and, seeing a puddle of water on the floor, asked loudly "Who wet the floor?" Pointing her finger at one woman, she inquired in an accusing voice, "Did you wet the floor?" Very embarrassed at being singled out as the culprit, the patient replied, "Why, no, it wasn't me." Staff frequently command patients in a parental voice: "Shut up!"; "Stay in your chair"; "Go to your place for lunch;" "I want you to go in and put on a dress, now get dressed!" and "Sit down, Grace." Such commands are often accompanied by

gestures, such as pointing a finger at the aged person, forcibly taking him [or her] by the arm, or "leading" him [or her] to a chair.

On some occasions, if patients do not comply, a threat is issued. Mrs. Garland, contrary to the directions of the activity director, repeatedly got up from her chair during a musical program. Later, the activity director asked one of the nurses, "What's the matter with Mrs. Garland today that she can't sit still?" The nurse explained the patient was anxious and agitated because her sons were away on vacation and had not been to visit. "Oh," replied the activity director, laughingly, "well, I told her if she didn't stay put, I would make her stand in the hall." (p. 39)

The activities that nursing home patients are expected to enjoy are ones that children love: birthday parties, and special outings to the zoo or amusement park (Shield, 1988). It is not unusual for nursing aides to act as if female patients are little girls. For example, some aides fix their hair in pigtails tied with ribbons and give them dolls (to which the aides refer as the patients' "babies") (Kimsey et al., 1981). Nursing aides often speak to their patients in baby talk. Such speech patterns have a detrimental effect on the self-esteem of the patients, convey less respect, and support dependent behavior. Nursing staff members who view patients as dependent also are more likely to use baby talk than those who do not (Pasupathi and Lockhenhoff, 2002).

Infantilization of nursing home patients includes patting patients on the head, calling them "baby," and addressing them by their first names without asking their preference. Researchers have found that those staff members who treated the patients as children were more likely to engage in psychologically abusive behavior than those who did not (Pillemer and Moore, 1989).

Name-Calling and Insulting

The most common types of psychological abuse reported by Pillemer and Moore (1989) and Foner (1994) were yelling at, swearing at, and insulting patients. Foner describes the behavior of Ms. Riley, a nursing aide at the home that she studied:

If looks could kill, hers would, and she often yelled in loud, cruel, and angry tones. "You better shut up or I'll fix your ass." "Eat your food," she screamed at a whining patient in the dayroom who was slow to eat. When a resident, in her own room, asked for a cup to spit into, Ms. Riley barked, "It's your spit, housekeeping will come to clean it up." As she left the room, Ms. Riley glared at the resident and said, with vehemence, "You bastard." To another complaining resident, Ms. Riley yelled, "I don't have to listen to you or look at you." . . . Sometimes groups of aides ganged up to tease a resident. One morning three aides were in the elevator with Mr. Langdon, an alert wheelchair-bound resident. They loudly laughed among themselves about how badly he smelled. "He needs a fire hose to clean him down," one commented. (1994, p. 41)

Depersonalization

Another type of psychological abuse is **depersonalization**—ignoring a patient or failing to communicate with him or her. For example:

On one occasion, Mrs. Garvey, a gentle 85-year-old woman, was sitting in the lounge; as a nurse aide walked by, Mrs. Garvey said, "Good morning." The aide did not reply. Another aide walked in and again Mrs. Garvey said, "Good morning." Again there was no reply. This scene occurred repeatedly; staff walked by as if she were not there. (Kayser-Jones, 1981)

It is not uncommon for patients to be treated as if they were nonpersons without an identity (for public opinion on the treatment of residents, see Exhibit 8.1). Shield (1988) gives the following illustration:

In the resident-care conference staff members are talking about a resident who is present. The resident is unable to hear what is being said because she is somewhat deaf. The resident interrupts the conversation and asks what is going on. Several staff members look surprised. In an exaggerated way, a staff member turns to face her, and speaks very slowly and loudly. After this statement, staff conversation returns to its previous quick-paced, low decibel level. (p. 197)

EXHIBIT 8.1. Survey Question Addressed to Public

Do you think the following is something that happens to almost all nursing home residents, many of them, some, or hardly any?

Residents are treated with dignity by the staff.

Almost all	Many	Some	Hardly any
14%	22%	46%	14%

Source: The NewsHour with Jim Lehrer/Kaiser Family Foundation/Harvard School of Public Health National Survey on Nursing Homes, September 2001.

SOME EFFECTS OF PSYCHOLOGICAL ABUSE

Depression

One of the most frequent emotional disorders of older persons is **depression.** It occurs with varying degrees of intensity and duration. Depression is so diverse in its symptoms that it is easily confused with other conditions, such as dementia. Depressive periods are often a pathological response to the loss of a significant person, unresolved grief, or anger. In addition, depression may result from nonphysical and physical abuse. Elderly nursing home patients may feel dehumanized because of the demeaning manner in which they are treated. This may result in the loss of self-esteem, autonomy, dignity, and interest in living (Sengstock and Steiner, 1996; Osgood et al., 1991).

Severe depression is the leading cause of suicide in late life. Some depressed older people commit suicide by slow, indirect means, such as not taking their medicine or by self-starvation. The following case of a nursing home patient illustrates this situation:

A frail elderly man in a nursing home who was deeply depressed repeatedly asked for a gun. He had made up his mind that he did not want to live any longer. Finally, knowing that he was a diabetic, he stopped eating. The staff ignored his fasting and continued giving him insulin shots until he lapsed into a diabetic coma and died.

Research done by Osgood and colleagues (1991) revealed that factors related to suicidal behavior in nursing homes include staff turnover and the size of the home. For instance, they found that homes with a staff turnover rate of 50 percent or higher yearly reported more cases of suicidal behavior among patients than those with a staff turnover of less than 10 percent. Also, nursing homes with more than 100 patients had a higher percentage of suicidal behavior than those with fewer patients. In addition, the researchers noted that patients who

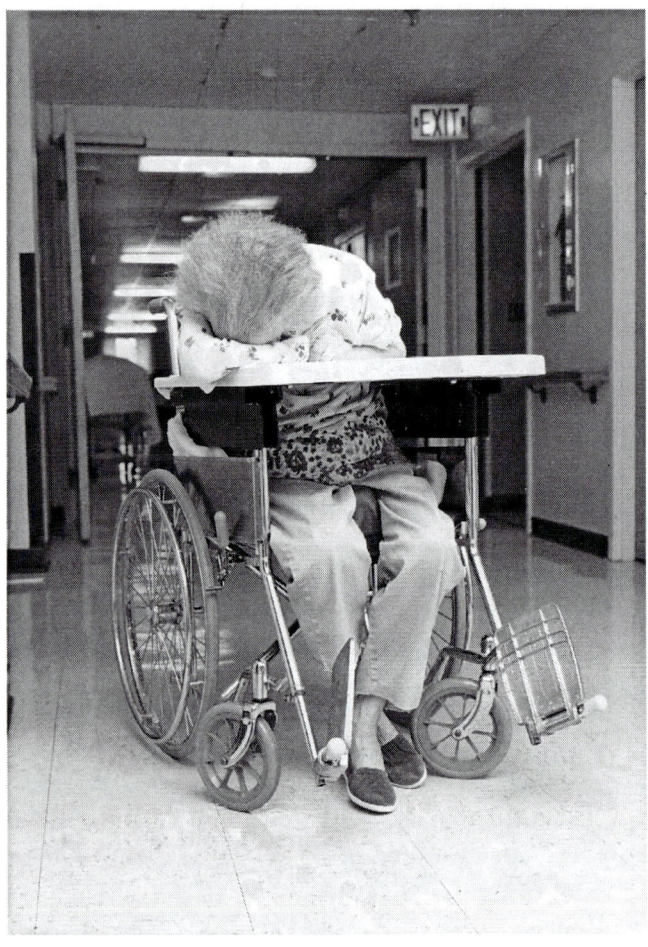

Depression.

lived in nursing homes with rigid policies that curtailed their autonomy and privacy tended to be at greater risk for suicidal behavior. Finally, suicidal behavior occurred in about 20 percent of the 463 homes that they studied.

Learned Helplessness

A major response of nursing home patients to psychological abuse is **learned helplessness,** a term coined by Seligman (1975). It may be defined as a fatalistic, passive attitude of accepting whatever comes along and a belief that all is hopeless (Harris, 1988). Patients begin to believe that events are beyond their control and that nothing can be done to change them. In such situations, they give up, become apathetic, and are resigned to their fate. In a total institution such as a nursing home, "learned helplessness is probably more pervasive than seen anywhere else in the human social environment" (Soloman, 1983).

Negative labeling is prevalent in nursing homes. Patients are often viewed by the staff as being dependent, powerless, and incompetent. This creates and reinforces the "learned helplessness" response in them and leads to even greater levels of dependency. Once patients are labeled in this way, they are then given less to do and less responsibility for their own care. For example, if the staff labels patients as being incompetent and dependent, then they will treat them as if they are. Those patients who accept such negative labeling learn to act even more dependent, and previous skills of independence are gradually lost. Finally, over time, they begin to think of themselves as incompetent and dependent, setting the stage for the vicious cycle of increasing incompetence and dependence. In other words, the label eventually proves to be a **self-fulfilling prophecy**.

Psychiatric Disorders

The maltreatment of nursing home patients in some cases may be severe enough to lead to post-traumatic stress disorder:

> This is an anxiety disorder in which severe psychological stress leads first to feelings of intense fear, terror, and helplessness, and then to a symptomatic state in which individuals are repeat-

edly disabled by recurring reminders and memories of the traumatic event. People with post-traumatic stress disorders avoid stimuli or people associated with the trauma and show symptoms of increased arousal, such as insomnia, irritability, and increased vigilance. (Booth et al., 1996)

NEGLECT

Psychological neglect refers to leaving persons alone for long periods of time without social stimulation. Pillemer and Moore (1989) found that in their study of the abuse of nursing home patients, 23 percent of the staff reported that they had observed the inappropriate isolation of patients. Patients singled out for isolation are often those who have been negatively labeled by the staff as aggressive. Their disruptive and unruly behavior is simply attributed to their bad temperament (with no accounting for underlying causes). Meddaugh (1993) examined psychological abuse in nursing homes by assessing the interactions between the patients and the staff. She found that certain patients, especially those that were considered aggressive, were excluded from group activities and rehabilitative efforts because the staff felt that they did not act in a way that was acceptable. She reports that many of the aggressive patients were left alone without social stimulation for long periods of time. Meddaugh (1993) cites the following two cases to illustrate psychological neglect:

> Mr. E was fed breakfast in bed and then left in bed. A couple of hours later his 20-minute daily care was given with little conversation. He usually was lifted out of bed until lunchtime where he sat beside the room window looking out on a brick wall. After lunch, which he usually refused, he was left again until it was time to return him to bed at 2:30 p.m. Until he had dinner at 7:00 p.m., Mr. E lay in a darkened room in complete silence.

> Mrs. U was taken to the TV room, where she sat in her gerichair for hours weeping. She did not look at the TV that was left on for her to watch. She stayed in this room, generally alone, until a caregiver returned her to bed. (p. 32)

These examples of psychological neglect are some of the cruelest types of punishment. Extended social isolation, for most people, is intolerable. Human beings are social animals and as such are dependent on one another. Our interaction with others is necessary for our survival and the satisfaction of our needs.

Chapter 9

Reducing the Risk of Physical and Psychological Abuse

Should criminals work as aides in nursing homes? As shocking as the thought of hiring criminals to take care of vulnerable, frail elderly patients may seem, it happens more often than one would think. "We've seen nursing homes where over a third of the nursing assistants had criminal records" (Pillemer et al., 2001, p. 32).

SCREENING PRACTICES

Although employee screening to identify potentially abusive personnel is a strong deterrent to patient maltreatment, it does not guarantee that abuse will not occur. Careful supervision of nursing aides after employment will help weed out those who may have slipped through the initial screening process. In this way, they will be identified and stopped before they can abuse other patients (Ramsey-Klawsnik, 2000).

Screening may include local, state, and Federal Bureau of Investigation criminal background checks as well as employee reference checks (see Table 9.1). Because most criminal background checks are performed by state and local law enforcement officials, they are usually only statewide and do not give patients all the protection that they need. As a result, a nursing aide that is fired from one facility for abuse can go to another state and obtain employment in a nursing home. Nationwide background checks by the FBI can be done if nursing homes request them. Although these checks could identify abusive nursing home employees elsewhere, few states use them. In some states, background checks are not given to all nursing home employees but only to those who provide direct patient care. Employees

TABLE 9.1. Some Types of Background Screening Mechanisms

Basic screening practices	Employee screening practices
Local criminal record check	Employment reference checks
State criminal record check	Personal reference checks
FBI criminal record check	Personal interviews
	Confirmation of education
Nursing aide registry record check	A written application

Source: Adapted from U.S. Department of Justice (1998).

who work in maintenance, housekeeping, and laundry services are excluded from screening.

In checking employment references, screening is made more difficult by the fact that previous employers usually will not divulge any information about a former worker (such as past abusive behaviors) for fear of defamation or other lawsuits. However, the prospective employer may obtain this information by getting written consent from the job applicant for its release. Careful screening should also include verifying the truthfulness of the information supplied by the applicant. Such checks will help reveal applicants who are lying or giving misleading information. Employment or educational histories with appreciable gaps may be a clue to problematic behavior or incarceration. Finally, conducting personal interviews that probe for in-depth information supplies the interviewer with information that may not be available through other screening techniques.

State survey agencies also play a role in preventing homes from hiring potentially abusive caregivers through the state's nursing aide registries. Federal law mandates that each state maintain a registry of nursing aides who have successfully completed an approved nurse aide training and competency program in that state. Before hiring an aide, homes must check the registry to verify that the aide has passed a competency evaluation. Aides whose names are not listed on the state's registry may work for up to four months in a nursing home to complete their training and pass the evaluation. The registry also includes convictions and documented evidence regarding patient abuse in that state. Nursing homes are required to check with the registry as part of the background screening process for prospective employees.

If a state survey agency determines that a nursing aide is responsible for abuse or theft of a patient's property, this information must be added to the state's nursing aide registry. Before employing an aide, homes are required to check with the registry to determine if the aide is in good standing and ensure that the aide is not banned from being employed in a nursing home.

However, states' nursing aide registries are not as effective as they could be because of problems in verifying accusations of abuse as well as the delays in posting this information. The delays between the time the state survey agencies learn that a nursing aide allegedly abused a patient to the date of the agencies' final determinations place nursing home patients in a vulnerable position to be further abused. For example one aide was charged with involuntary manslaughter when an 89-year-old blind, invalid woman drowned after being left in a bathtub.

> It took seven months for the worker's name to be placed on a list of aides who have abused or neglected patients. During this time, the same nursing aide beat a 91-year-old woman after she resisted being helped into bed. (Chan, 2002)

Although the Centers for Medicare and Medicaid Services (CMS) require nursing home officials to notify the state survey agency of allegations of abuse in their facilities immediately, often nursing home officials are not prompt in doing so, according to an investigation completed in 2002 by the Government Accounting Office (GAO). Abuse reports in three states—Illinois, Georgia, and Pennsylvania—were studied by the GAO. Of the 158 cases of alleged physical and sexual abuse that they reviewed, 105 involved nursing aides. Table 9.2 reveals that twenty-seven of the forty-one aides had their registry files annotated. Some determinations took ten months or longer. Such delayed reporting of abuse allegations leaves the patients in a vulnerable position as well as compromises the available evidence. In addition, it is not unusual for witnesses in criminal cases to have poor recall with the passage of time, which in turn hinders the investigation.

Even more troubling is that the abuse of nursing home patients frequently goes unreported and ignored. Some reasons for this include the following:

- Nursing home personnel and the patients' families may not believe the patients when they say that they have been abused.
- Sometimes family members are afraid that the patient will be asked to leave the home if they complain.
- Employees may not want to "blow the whistle" on a fellow co-worker when they see him or her abusing a patient.
- The nursing home administrator is concerned about the home getting bad publicity or a poor reputation.
- Patients may be afraid to tell anyone about their maltreatment because of fear of retaliation.

For tips on reporting suspected abuse, see Exhibit 9.1.

TABLE 9.2. Cases of Alleged Abuse Involving Nursing Aides in Three States

State	Cases involving nursing aides (1999)	Aides notified of intent to annotate registry records	Aides whose registry records were annotated (2002)
Georgia	31	9	5
Illinois	40	27	22
Pennsylvania	34	5	0
Total	105	41	27

Source: United States General Accounting Office (2002).

EXHIBIT 9.1. Reporting Suspected Abuse in Nursing Homes

1. Contact the state survey agency.
2. Go to the nursing home administrator.
3. Call the long-term care ombudsman.
4. Contact adult protective services, law enforcement, or the state licensing agency.

Remember that the situation could get worse and the patient could be seriously injured. The person who is being abusive is probably abusing other patients as well.

Source: Adapted from The Center for Advocacy for the Rights and Interests of the Elderly (CARIE). (1999). Competence with compassion: An abuse prevention training program for long-term care staff. Philadelphia, PA: CARIE, p. 40.

STAFF EDUCATION AND TRAINING

Maltreatment of patients appears to be in part a response to the nursing aides' stressful working conditions, which, as we have previously mentioned, include being understaffed, undersupervised, and undertrained. Because nursing aides have the most contact with patients, providing them with abuse prevention training is one of the best approaches in dealing with the problem of abuse. "Training is the only way staff will know: what exactly constitutes abuse; what is expected of them with regards to abuse; and what their facility's policies and procedure are" (Pillemer et al., 2001, p. 45).

One of the most well-known training programs, "Competence with Compassion: An Abuse Prevention Training Program for Long-Term Care Staff" was developed by Beth Hudson for The Center for Advocacy for the Rights and Interests of the Elderly (CARIE) (Pillemer and Hudson, 1993; Keller, 1996). This program, which began in 1989, has three main goals: (1) to increase staff awareness of abuse, neglect, and potential abuse in any setting where people are dependent upon others for assistance; (2) to equip staff with appropriate conflict intervention strategies so abuse can be avoided; and (3) to reduce incidences of abuse, thus improving the quality of life for both the person who requires care and the caregiver. To accomplish these goals, this innovative program consists of a seven-module training manual (see Table 9.3) as well as overheads, handouts, and an award-winning video, *At the End of the Day*.

A pretest-posttest instrument administered by CARIE staff was used to provide information on the outcome of the program. The data revealed a drop in abuse observed by aides and a significant reduction in the amount of patient-staff conflict. The aides also reported a notable decrease in burnout.

Another abuse prevention training package developed for nursing home aides is "Who's Abusing Who?" This program incorporates the stories of paraprofessionals and their suggestions for managing stress "so we don't take it out on others." It is comprised of a twelve-minute video drama and a twelve-page booklet. "The training appeared to increase job satisfaction, which has been shown to lower stress and frustration, and this in turn may help to lower the incidence of elder abuse in nursing homes" (Braun et al., 1997, p. 13).

TABLE 9.3. CARIE Abuse Prevention Program Training Modules

Module	Purpose
I. Introduction	To introduce the trainer, the philosophy of the training, and the key goals of the workshop
II. A Look at the Work	To start the group thinking about the challenges of being a professional caregiver and to identify the potential for abuse in the context of professional caregiving
III. What Is Abuse?	To provide participants with definitions of abuse, indicators, and information about how to report suspected abuse and neglect
IV. Why Abuse?	To raise awareness of the ways in which abuse is not necessarily the act of malicious or criminal people but can occur in daily situations with caregivers who may mean no intentional harm
V. A Case Scenario	To analyze an incident of suspected abuse from a variety of perspectives, exploring the complex nature of stress, frustration, and conflict, using the video *At the End of the Day*
VI. Conflict Management	To provide an opportunity for participants to learn and practice strategies and interventions to help cope with difficult situations
VII. Wrap-up and Evaluation	To review the topics covered in the workshop, reinforce main points, and provide opportunity for feedback from participants

Source: The Center for Advocacy for the Rights and Interests of the Elderly (CARIE). (1999). Competence with compassion: An abuse prevention training program for long-term care staff. Philadelphia, PA: CARIE. Reprinted with permission. Additional information about this training program can be obtained online at <www.carie.org>.

A third program, "Working It Out: Support Groups for Nursing Assistants" (Wilner, 1994), which includes a video and a leader's notebook, was designed to reduce stress and turnover among nursing aides by conducting support groups for them. The most often discussed subjects that emerged from the group included problems in communicating with fellow workers and supervisors, being understaffed, and managing difficult residents. Group members reported improved communication skills after participation in the support group and modest reductions in turnover rates were found. The directors believed that the program had also helped prevent occurrences of the verbal abuse that often arises when tensions increase.

Finally, *Nursing Assistant Monthly* (Frontline Publishing) is a subscription-based continuing education program for nursing aides that features in-service training modules. It goes beyond the technical aspects of training by addressing such topics as managing resident conflict, dementia care, and working with residents' family members. The program newsletter is sent every month to each nursing aide in a participating facility. In addition, the facility receives a monthly facilitator's guide. *Nursing Assistant Monthly* has developed a unique model for the training and professional development of nursing aides, which helps to build self-esteem and professionalism.

ADVOCACY

The nationwide long-term care ombudsman program, mandated through the 1978 amendments to the **Older Americans Act,** requires each state to have a long-term care ombudsperson who is responsible for identifying, investigating, and resolving complaints of nursing home patients, as well as those in other residential care facilities such as board-and-care homes and assisted living facilities. Ombudsperson responsibilities also include:

- furnishing information to patients and residents about long-term care services;
- representing the interests of patients and residents before governmental agencies;
- educating and informing consumers and the public about issues and concerns related to long-term care;
- helping to encourage the participation of citizen organizations in the program; and
- guarding the rights and well-being of patients and residents. (These rights include protecting them from neglect and abuse.)

In a recent case of verbal abuse, the ombudsman met with the administrator and the director of nursing at the facility on behalf of the resident. After several meetings, the offending staff person was identified and transferred to another unit. The ombudsman continues to visit the resident who made the complaints and other residents within the facility and also attends resident council meetings to remain on the alert for other such problems. (Menio and Keller, 2000)

Most regular visits to nursing homes are made by ombudsman volunteers, who are often referred to as the "foot soldiers" of long-term care. They are trained to assist the ombudsman. In 2001, about 13,700 volunteers served in homes throughout the nation. The volunteers bring a positive community presence into nursing homes, helping to improve the facility's quality of care and the patient's quality of life.

PART IV:
FRAUD, REFORM,
AND RECOMMENDATIONS

Chapter 10

Exploitation of Nursing Home Patients: Their Finances and Rights

The administrator of a nursing home developed a close relationship with and won the confidence of about a half-dozen private-pay patients (those patients responsible for the entire cost of their care). She offered to manage their money because their relatives lived far away. The patients gladly accepted her offer. Over time, the nursing home administrator wrote a number of checks to herself and bilked the patients out of thousands of dollars.

When the term **exploitation** is used in the context of elder mistreatment in nursing homes, it is usually one of two types. The first type, **financial abuse,** involves the theft or misuse of a patient's money by others. Financial abuse differs from the outright theft of a patient's possessions in that it is often the result of a betrayal of trust, as in the example just given. It is an insidious crime that tends to consist of a pattern of behavior rather than a single incident (Wilbur and Reynolds, 1996). A second type of abuse that we will focus on in this chapter is the violation of a nursing home patient's rights. For example, allowing nursing home personnel to make decisions for cognitively alert patients instead of giving the patients a right to decide for themselves is a violation of federal law.

FINANCIAL ABUSE

Financial abuse in nursing homes usually results from fraudulent practices by nursing home employees or mismanagement by administrators and nursing home owners. About two decades ago the United States Government Accounting Office (GAO) investigated reports of wide-scale fraud involving patients' finances. They conducted an audit of thirty homes in six states. The GAO found that each of the thirty homes had failed to safeguard patients' funds in several ways. Shortages were found in patients' accounts, and medical supplies and services were being improperly charged to them. In some cases, the funds of dead or transferred patients were retained by the homes (Moss and Halamandaris, 1977). Today, financial abuse is one of the fastest growing categories of crimes against persons in nursing homes because a significant number of nursing home patients are unable to prevent it, or even know that they are being victimized.

Trust Accounts

One of the most common types of financial abuse in nursing homes is the embezzlement of patients' **trust accounts** (also called personal allowances). Medicaid patients receive a small monthly allowance, which can be spent any way they choose. It is generally used for such purposes as haircuts, clothing, candy, newspapers, and cigarettes. The facility, if requested, will maintain trust accounts for Medicaid patients as well as for private-pay patients so that they do not need to keep money in their rooms. The following cases are examples of theft involving patients' trust accounts:

> A bookkeeper in a nursing home who was in control of the patients' trust accounts began inappropriately manipulating the nursing home's financial records. She embezzled over about $75,000 from patients' trust accounts by making withdrawals at automatic teller machines and altering records to hide her crime. In another home, a bookkeeper embezzled over $33,000 from nursing home funds and patients' trust accounts. (Hodge, 1998)

> A social services aide . . . admitted to using money from the patients' trust fund[s] to buy clothing and other personal items, then returning and exchanging them for merchandise for herself. The crime was discovered after a Wal-Mart employee contacted the nursing home about frequent returns made without a receipt. ("Woman Pleads Guilty," 2001)

Bank Accounts

Another type of financial abuse is obtaining access to and using patients' bank accounts. Mentally impaired patients are often the victims of this type of abuse.

> A former administrator of a nursing home gained access to the bank accounts of two Alzheimer's patients who were unable to handle their own finances. He transferred $68,000 of their funds to pay off his personal debts. (Schlichter, 2000)

In another case, a nursing home official stole money from a deceased patient's bank accounts.

> A former admissions director stole thousands of dollars from a patient *after* the patient died. The director said that she obtained power of attorney for a 78-year-old woman after her death at the nursing home . . . she forged the woman's name on bank signature cards to get access to her checking and savings accounts. (Munz, 2001b, p. 8)

Improper Charges for Services and Drugs

This scheme involves charging the patient's families or the state for services never performed, services not medically authorized, or therapy never given. Other fraudulent activities include charging for drugs not provided, billing for brand-name drugs but dispensing generic substitutions, and charging for the prescribed quantity of drugs but dispensing a lesser amount or lesser strength to the patient.

Identity Theft

Identity theft refers to the wrongful acquisition and use of one's personal data in a fraudulent manner for financial gain. These thieves prey on nursing home patients by ripping out checks from the middle of their checkbooks, stealing their credit cards, or using their Social Security number to apply for loans, credit, and phone service.

In one instance, a ring of identity thieves stole more than $20,000 from an elderly woman in a nursing home by writing checks from her bank account. In another case, a nursing aide and her boyfriend used a patient's identity to get telephone service and attempted to illegally obtain a credit card (Elrick, 2000). Identity theft is a growing problem among nursing home patients (and the general public). According to one law enforcement officer, nursing home patients are the ideal victims; no one is likely to know when their personal information was taken, and often patients may be too mentally and physically impaired to protect such information. He noted that nursing homes should help their patients by guarding critical personal information such as their Social Security numbers, which are regularly used as identifiers. They are often on patients' charts, which are available to employees and even visitors (Burns, 2000).

REFORM OF NURSING HOME REGULATIONS

The landmark passage of OBRA (1987) contained a major reform of nursing home regulations, improved the quality-of-care standards for nursing homes that participate in the Medicare and Medicaid programs, and strengthened federal and state supervision. These reforms grew out of the failure of the Reagan administration to deregulate the nursing home industry. This failure resulted in a study of nursing home regulations by the National Academy of Sciences, Institute of Medicine (IOM). The results of this study led to OBRA '87, which brought about sweeping changes in how the quality of care in nursing homes is defined and measured. In addition, it revised the inspection process, enforcement system, and standards of nursing home care. Homes that fail to comply with any federal provisions are faced with the loss of Medicare and Medicaid certification. Because a large proportion of a nursing home's revenue is supplied by some form of federal reimbursement, such a loss could be financially devastating. However, even with these reform measures an unacceptable number of homes continue to provide poor quality of care.

Federal provisions, as quoted from OBRA '87, require that every nursing home "care for its residents in such a manner and in such an environment as will promote maintenance or enhancement of the quality of life of each resident." In addition, the law requires each nursing facility to "provide services and activities to attain or maintain for each patient the highest practical physical, mental, and psychological well-being." Emphasis is placed on dignity, choice, and self-determination for nursing home patients. The following are some of the major rights of nursing home patients as mandated by OBRA '87 (adapted from Burger et al., 2000; National Citizens' Coalition for Nursing Home Reform 2001a; AARP, 1991).

I. The Right to the Security of Possessions and Finances
  A. The patient has the right to the security of his or her possessions, including the right to manage his or her own financial affairs, file a complaint with the state survey and certification agency for abuse, neglect, or misappropriation of his or her property if the nursing home is handling his or her financial affairs.
  B. The nursing home cannot require patients to deposit their personal funds with them. If the home accepts written responsibility for patients' funds it must keep funds over $50 in an interest-bearing account and do a complete and separate accounting of each resident's funds, with a written record of all transactions.
  C. The nursing home cannot charge, solicit, accept, or receive gifts, money, donations, or other considerations as a precondition for admission or continued stay for persons eligible for Medicaid.
  D. The nursing home must not charge a patient for any item or service covered by Medicaid, specifically including routine personal hygiene items and services.
II. Abuse and Restraint Rights
  A. The patient has the right to be free from physical or mental abuse, corporal punishment, and involuntary seclusion as well as any physical and chemical restraints used for purposes of discipline or convenience of the staff rather than the well-being of the patient.
  B. Restraints should be used only under a physician's written orders to treat the patients' medical symptoms and to ensure their safety and the safety of others.
  C. Patients have the right to refuse treatment, including restraints.

D. Psychopharmacologic medication can be given only if ordered by a physician.

III. The Right to Privacy and Confidentiality
  A. The patient has the right to participate in social, religious, and community activities as he or she chooses.
  B. The patient has the right to privacy in medical treatment, personal visits, telephone communications, and confidentiality of personal and clinical records. Patients' mail must not be opened without their consent.
  C. Personal and clinical records should be kept confidential.
  D. The patient has the right to private and unrestricted communication with any person of their choice.

IV. The Right to Make Independent Decisions
  A. The right to choose their own physician.
  B. The right to vote.
  C. The right to participate in a resident council.
  D. The right to participate in community activities, both inside and outside the nursing home.
  E. The right to reasonable accommodation of their needs and preferences by the facility.

V. The Right to Visits
  A. Immediate visits by the patient's relatives with the patient's consent.
  B. Reasonable visits by organizations or individuals providing health, social, legal, or other services, subject to a patient's consent.
  C. Immediate access by a patient's personal physician and representatives from the state survey agency and ombudsman programs.
  D. The right for an ombudsman to review a patient's clinical records with the patient's permission.

VI. Right to Information
  A. The patients have the right to have a copy of the nursing home's rules and regulations, including a written copy of their rights.
  B. The patient must be informed in advance of any plans to change his or her room or roommate.
  C. Patients have the right to daily communication in their language.

    D. Assistance is to be provided if the patient has a sensory impairment.
VII. Rights During Transfers and Discharges
    A. The right to remain in the nursing home unless a transfer is necessary for the patient's welfare, the patient no longer needs nursing home care, to protect the health and safety of the staff or other patients, and for nonpayment of stay.
    B. The patient must receive a thirty-day notice of transfer or discharge.
    C. The nursing home must sufficiently prepare for a safe transfer or discharge of the patient.
VIII. The Right to Complain
    A. The right to present grievances to the staff of the nursing home, or to any other person without fear of reprisal.
    B. Prompt efforts should be made by the home to resolve grievances.
    C. The right to complain to the state survey agency and ombudsman program.

Why Are There Patients' Rights?

The nursing home is an institution, with institutional bureaucracy and management. Residents are physically frail and often mentally confused. These factors help explain why the law places so much emphasis on patients' rights. (Burger et al., 2000)

    In summary, patients in nursing homes have the right to the security of their possessions and finances and to be free from physical or mental abuse as well as physical and chemical restraints used for purposes of discipline or convenience. They have the right to privacy and confidentiality and to make their own decisions. Finally, each patient is entitled to visits, information about the home, and to voice their grievances free from fear of retaliation.

Chapter 11

Summary and Conclusions

The term *nursing home* often carries negative connotations in everyday speech. It conjures up a host of images and descriptions, including "warehouse for the elderly" and "place where the elderly are undergoing slow euthanasia." As a result, many persons are adamant about not going to a nursing home. For example:

> "I would rather just drop dead—that's the way I feel about a nursing home," said [an 84-year-old woman], who worked in nursing homes for her job with a sitting service earlier in life. "I've been there, not as a patient, but I've been there to take care of a patient and I know. . . . I figure sooner or later I might have to go in a nursing home, but they'll take me out of here kicking and screaming, I'll tell you." (Nelson, 2001, p. E1)*

One reason for the negative image that people have of nursing homes is the fear that they could be abused. This fear is not without justification. According to some researchers, "abuse, although often not detected or reported, in fact, existed in every facility we have surveyed. It is a serious problem" (Pillemer et al., 2001, p. 32).

A national telephone survey of 1,309 randomly selected adults was conducted by the NewsHour with Jim Lehrer (2001). They investigated the public's attitudes toward nursing homes. When the respondents were asked about their willingness to move into a nursing home, 43 percent said, "I would find it totally unacceptable," whereas 47 percent replied, "I would not like it, but would probably come to accept it." Only 10 percent said, "I would accept it as being the best thing for me." Two-thirds of the respondents reported that they be-

---

*Reprinted by permission of the Knoxville News-Sentinel Company.

lieved the staff abuses at least *some* patients, and they also said that only some or hardly any patients could rely on their personal belongings to be safe.

The survey's findings further reveal that 60 percent of the respondents believed nursing homes provide an important service in offering affordable, round-the-clock care. However, a significant majority (80 percent) thought that nursing homes are understaffed, and two-thirds believe that nursing home staff members are poorly trained.

This book has attempted to outline the major types of patient abuse in nursing homes. In this final chapter, we will summarize some of these problems along with recommendations for helping nursing homes create a safer and more abuse-free environment.

1. Although careful hiring practices are no guarantee that an undesirable person or one with a criminal background will not be hired, it does cut down on the chances of it happening.

Recommendation: Administrators should screen prospective employees by checking references, conducting criminal background checks, ensuring thorough interviews, and consulting their state registries before hiring employees. As we noted earlier, each state is required by law to have a registry of nursing aides. This registry contains information on any finding of abuse or misappropriation of property concerning nursing home patients in their state. However, a system is needed by which states can share information about known abusers so workers cannot evade these registries by moving from state to state. Furthermore, a federal law is needed that requires *national* criminal background checks of those persons working in nursing homes.

2. Generally, nursing aides, who constitute the largest proportion of workers in nursing homes and provide most of the direct care to patients, do not receive the training they need. They receive minimum training for providing personal care services as well as dealing with a variety of interpersonal problems, which they encounter on a daily basis.

Recommendation: In our national survey of nursing homes, the fact that approximately 60 percent of those who self-reported theft were nursing aides is not surprising; nursing aides have more access to patients and their possessions than do those in other occupational positions. However, differential access alone is not sufficient to explain abuse. Those who self-reported abuse tended to have more conflict with patients as well as more negative attitudes toward them.

Two types of prevention programs should be made available to nursing aides. First, a program such as "Competence with Compassion" (see Chapter 8) to equip the aides with conflict intervention strategies and to help them develop more favorable attitudes toward their patients is needed. Second, a program to teach *all* the employees in the home about the importance of respecting patients' belongings and understanding the sentimental value that they attach to them would be beneficial (see Chapter 5).

3. To provide good quality of care in nursing homes, facilities need to provide staff sufficient training. They also need sufficient numbers of staff members to care for the patients. Research reveals that the physical and psychological abuse of patients are closely related to the stressful working conditions in nursing homes due in part to the inadequate staffing levels and high turnover rates (see Chapter 2).

Recommendation: Current staffing levels of some homes are not adequate to provide quality care to patients. A recent report of the Centers for Medicare and Medicaid Services (2002) to Congress stated that nursing homes with a low ratio of nursing personnel to patients were more likely to provide substandard care. A minimum staffing ratio of 4.1 hours of direct, one-on-one care per day was recommended.

4. Nearly 20 percent (19.3 percent) of the respondents in our study suspected their co-workers of stealing from patients, whereas 6 percent actually reported seeing them steal. They were asked what they did about it when they saw or suspected an employee of stealing. About 60 percent said that they reported it to their supervisor. In most cases the employees said that either nothing was done or they were not sure of the outcome.

Recommendation: All cases of suspected abuse must be reported and *promptly* investigated. This sends a clear message to the staff that abuse will not be tolerated. Delayed reporting of abuse allegations compromises the available evidence and could leave the patient in a vulnerable position. An employee that reports any type of actual or suspected mistreatment of patients should be informed (by his or her supervisor or the management) of the action taken by the home. By ignoring such reports and not doing anything about them, the administration sends a message to its employees that it does not care about the mistreatment of patients. This attitude only leads to more abusive behavior.

5. All organizations have systems of social control to ensure that their members generally behave in expected and approved ways. This control can be exercised formally either by management or the criminal justice system, and informally through the reactions of co-workers. These reactions could include disapproval, criticism, and ostracism.

When we asked our respondents what they thought would happen to them if they were caught stealing from patients, 86.4 percent believed they would be fired; only 42.4 percent believed they would be reported to the police. Because most nursing home administrators would rather fire employees than prosecute them, nursing home employees are usually not worried about facing legal action.

Recommendation: Research reveals that informal social controls initiated by one's co-workers are often more effective in stopping deviance than formal actions are (Hollinger and Clark, 1983). A nursing home administrator that we interviewed pointed out that, if possible, she preferred that the aides work in pairs so that they could "keep an eye on each other." Also, she found that having employees leave together or in groups at shift changes was a deterrent to theft. While visiting a nursing home one morning, one of the authors overheard an aide talking to another aide who had just yelled and sworn at a patient. The aide told the abusive employee that she found such behavior unacceptable, as did the nursing home, and that she had better change her attitude or she would be fired.

6. About 40 percent of the employees in our study perceived that their chances of being detected stealing patients' property was "very unlikely" or "somewhat unlikely." These findings indicate the ease with which many employees believe they can steal and reflect the lack of security that prevails in nursing homes today.

Recommendation: Nursing home management should attempt to win the cooperation and involvement of all the staff members in helping to make the home more secure. This process should begin at the time a new employee is hired. New employees should be required to complete the training programs previously discussed. Employees should be motivated to be aware of potential abuse incidents and to report suspicious persons and unusual behavior. In this way, the staff becomes a valuable asset and partner in abuse prevention.

In conclusion, we can no longer allow this national tragedy of abuse in nursing homes to persist. It continues to plague one of the most vulnerable and frail segments of our population. We must meet this challenge by understanding this pervasive problem and conceiving effective strategies to deal with it. We have the capability to stop it. It is time we do.

Appendix

Methodology

Two primary methods for studying deviance in organizations exist: the **ethnographic study** and the self-report survey. In the ethnographic study approach, the researcher typically spends a considerable amount of time observing the organization's routines and talking to its members. This approach produces an in-depth grasp of the organization and a rich description of how it works. Skilled ethnographers can penetrate the inner workings of an organization and uncover much that may not be readily apparent to casual observers.

The second major approach to studying deviance in organizational settings is the self-report survey. This technique has been adapted from criminology, in which it is often used to study juvenile delinquency and crime. In a self-report study, a sample of individuals is given a questionnaire and asked to "self-report" on their deviant activities and to provide other relevant information about themselves. The questionnaire is confidential and the participants remain anonymous. Clearly, to ask participants in a study to self-report on activities such as theft or other forms of deviant behavior is a sensitive matter, and the validity of such reports is never perfect. For obvious reasons, respondents often underreport their activities or refuse to participate at all. Despite these potential problems, self-reports have long been regarded as a reliable method for studying delinquent behavior and crime (Lab and Allen, 1984; Hindelang et al., 1981). Hollinger and Clark (1983) successfully used the self-report survey to investigate employee theft in retail and manufacturing industries and hospitals.

To investigate the problem of theft from nursing home patients, we used both the self-report survey and the ethnographic case study. First, we surveyed nursing home employees, administrators, and the family members of patients. We then supplemented the survey data with site visits to six nursing homes, where we interviewed patients, employees, administrators, and some family members.

DATA COLLECTION

With funding from the Retirement Research Foundation, we surveyed employees, administrators, and family members of patients in forty-seven nursing homes in 1997 and 1998. The homes were carefully selected to represent different regions of the country and different types of homes. We started by identifying the ten states with the largest elderly populations (California, Florida, Illinois, Massachusetts, Michigan, New York, Ohio, Pennsylvania, Texas, and Wisconsin). These states account for approximately half of the nation's elderly population and are geographically diverse. Next we used the 1997 Directory of Nursing Homes. This directory lists almost all nursing homes in the country and provides information on their location, administrators, size, and type. Small homes were defined as those with fewer than fifty beds, medium-sized homes with between fifty and 199 beds, and large homes had 200 or more beds. Then, we grouped the homes according to size and type of ownership into six categories (small nonprofit, small profit, medium nonprofit, medium profit, large nonprofit, and large profit). Finally, we randomly selected 100 homes from the list of homes based roughly on their proportional representation among nursing homes nationwide. That is, we tried to select a group of homes that would be representative of the size and types of nursing homes across the nation.

To begin to solict homes to participate in our study, we selected fifty-two homes from our master list and contacted the administrators by telephone. We explained the nature of our study and invited them to participate. Homes that declined to participate were replaced by similar homes drawn from the master list. Although fifty-two homes agreed to participate in the study, some homes later withdrew from the project after it was too late to replace them. Thus, we had a final sample of forty-seven homes. The final sample does broadly represent nursing homes nationwide.

Typically in self-report studies, questionnaires are handed to or mailed directly to the participants by the researchers; that is the method we would have preferred to follow for our study. Unfortunately, based on prior work in nursing homes, we knew that many administrators would not feel at liberty to provide us with the names and addresses of their employees. We also knew that administrators would be even more unwilling to give us names and addresses of family members. Hence, we had to develop alternative ways to distribute our questionnaires.

When administrators agreed to participate in the study, we asked them how many employees they had, and how many patients with family members lived in the home. We then mailed them the appropriate number of survey packets for each group and asked the administrators to distribute them according to our instructions. Although it is less than perfect, this method was the only one open to us given our limited resources. For the employee questionnaires, we asked the administrators to give each employee a survey packet, which contained a copy of the questionnaire, a cover letter explaining the project and assuring the respondents that their answers would be confidential, and a business-return envelope. We suggested to administrators that the most convenient way to distribute the questionnaires would be to include them with the next employee paychecks, but homes were free to distribute our materials otherwise if they so desired. After six weeks, we contacted the homes again and asked them to distribute a second set of questionnaire packets to employees. By this means, we hoped to give those who may have missed out on the first mailing a second chance to participate. To learn more about the homes themselves, we sent a different questionnaire to the administrators that focused on personnel and security policies.

EMPLOYEE QUESTIONNAIRES

The questionnaire for employees was divided into different sections. We began by asking the respondents about their job title, hours worked, and the length of time they had been employed in the nursing home. An important question in this section concerned how often the employee went into patients' rooms as part of his or her job. On the basis of the routine activities theory (see Chapter 3), we assumed access to patients' rooms to be a prerequisite for theft. Hence, we asked respondents about how often, if ever, they enter patients' rooms and whether they typically work alone or with others. We hoped that these questions would help us better identify those who have the greatest opportunity to commit theft from patients.

Next, we asked a series of questions concerning job satisfaction, and attitudes toward supervisors and patients. We surmised that employees who are dissatisfied or unhappy with their work might be more likely to engage in theft from patients and other types of abuse. The questions regarding attitudes toward patients were designed to uncover whether employees liked or disliked their patients and how often patients behaved in a verbally or physically abusive manner toward them. As with the questions on general job satisfaction, our logic here was that employees who are in conflict with or who feel that they are being poorly treated by patients will be more likely to steal from them or otherwise abuse them in return.

The most sensitive part of the questionnaire concerned asking employees about their own theft from patients. Because theft is a deviant activity, it is difficult to measure it accurately. Often when an item disappears from a patient's room, it is not easy to determine whether it has simply been misplaced, inadvertently taken by another patient, or stolen by an employee or someone else (such as a visitor or a volunteer). The nursing home industry frequently responds to the issue of theft from patients with a form of scapegoating. Theft is often blamed on the patients themselves, who are accused of simply losing or misplacing items or of stealing from one another (Harris and Benson, 1998). Because about half of the patients in nursing homes suffer from dementia, they make ideal scapegoats.

When patients are caught with other people's belongings, the items usually are odd things of minor value. These items tend to turn up after a while and can be returned to their owners. However, research conducted by the authors suggests that the more valuable items that disappear from nursing home patients are not likely to return. Furthermore, the circumstances surrounding their disappearances suggest theft by deliberate criminal intent and not misguided kleptomania by demented patients.

MEASURING THEFT

In designing our measures of theft, we used several different approaches. We asked employees to report on theft by others as well as themselves, and we asked family members to report on the experiences of their relatives in nursing homes.

Our first approach to the problem of measuring theft was to ask employees about their observations of theft by others. We asked employees to report if in the past year they had seen someone, such as another patient, an employee, or a visitor, stealing from patients. Then we asked a series of follow-up questions about what item or items were stolen. The response categories were

1. money, credit cards, checks;
2. televisions, VCR;
3. jewelry;
4. clothing;
5. stamps;
6. food, candy, flowers;
7. knickknacks;
8. cosmetics, toiletries;
9. cigarettes or other tobacco products; and
10. other items.

We then asked for an estimate of the dollar value of the stolen items. Response categories ranged from "less than \$5" to "more than \$50."

Employees also were asked to tell us whether the most recent employee theft that they had observed had been reported to the nursing home, and if so, what action, if any, the nursing home had taken. Finally, we asked employees how likely it was that they would get caught if they stole something that belonged to a patient and, if they did get caught, what they thought would happen to them.

Our second approach was to ask employees to self-report on their own theft behavior. After reassuring them that their answers would be anonymous, we began by asking if in the past year they had taken something that did not belong to them from a patient's room. Those who answered "yes" were then asked the number of times they had taken something, what they had taken, and what the estimated dollar value of the item or items was.

After the section on theft was completed, employees were asked a short list of questions that were designed to provide us with information about the social characteristics of our respondents. Thus, we asked about sex, age, race, marital status, education, and household income. The information gained from these questions permitted us to learn more about who works in nursing homes and who is most likely to steal from patients.

RESPONSE RATES FROM THE SURVEY OF EMPLOYEES

We received completed questionnaires from 1,116 employees. Because we do not know how many questionnaires were actually distributed to employees, it is difficult to determine the response rate with certainty. Based on the total number of employees reported to us by administrators, we conservatively estimate that the response rate was approximately 22 percent. Although this rate is lower than ideal, it is quite similar to response rates reported by other nursing home researchers (e.g., Goergen, 2001). It is important to remember that a questionnaire on such a sensitive topic may threaten some employees, who may refuse to participate out of fear of exposure. Overall, we were not surprised at our response rate because in two smaller pilot studies that we had conducted earlier we received a similar response rate (Harris and Benson, 1997).

VICTIMIZATION SURVEY

As noted earlier, the self-report survey is a commonly used method for collecting data in criminology. Despite its popularity, however, it suffers from the understandable shortcoming that offenders may not tell the truth about their activities. Hence, criminologists, in looking for other sources of information about crime, have used another technique—the victimization survey. Victimization surveys are similar to self-report surveys in that they ask ordinary people about their experiences with crime. However, instead of asking whether the respondent has committed a crime, victimization surveys ask whether the respondent has been victimized by a particular crime within some given time period. To supplement what we learned about theft from employees, we decided to conduct a victimization survey in our sample of nursing homes.

Although victimization surveys can provide much useful information about criminal events, it is difficult to use this approach in nursing homes. All self-administered surveys require that the respondent be able to read and understand the questions and directions. Unfortunately, close to half of nursing home patients suffer from cognitive deficiencies and are incapable of completing self-administered surveys. In this situation, one option would be to administer surveys only to patients who are mentally capable of filling them out. We rejected this option for two reasons. First, ascertaining the mental capabilities of patients can be a complicated and time-consuming undertaking, which requires direct access to patients. We did not have the time or the resources to conduct these evaluations. Another reason for not surveying only mentally competent patients is that patients who are mentally incompetent some or all of the time may be the most vulnerable victims for thieves. Because of their disabilities, they are unable to protect themselves and their property. They may even be unable to ask others for help or to report any losses that they suffer. Hence, a victimization survey of only part of the population might grossly underestimate the true amount of victimization in nursing homes.

FAMILY MEMBERS' QUESTIONNAIRE

Nevertheless, it is important to try to get the victim's perspective on theft in nursing homes. Thus, we decided to ask family members of patients to serve as proxy respondents for their relatives. We assumed that family members have sufficient awareness of the possessions that patients have and will notice if items are missing. In addition, we assumed that patients themselves might be more likely to report theft to their family members than to nursing home personnel. Accordingly, we designed a questionnaire for family members that asked them to report on the experiences of their relatives.

Ideally, we would have liked to mail the family questionnaire to the families of all the patients in the nursing homes in our sample. However, most of the nursing homes in the sample did not feel at liberty to provide us with the names and addresses of the family members. They were concerned that doing so might violate family members' privacy. Hence, to distribute the family questionnaires, we provided each home with a display box for the questionnaire packets and a large sign that invited family members to participate in the study. We asked the nursing home administrators to place the box in a conspicuous location in the home (for example, near the main entrance in the lobby of the home) and use whatever means they could to encourage families to participate in the study. The family packets contained a copy of the questionnaire, a cover letter, and a business-return envelope. A total of 417 surveys were completed and returned to us.

The family questionnaire began by asking the family member to specify how they were related to the patient. Next, we asked how long the patient had been in the nursing home and how often the family member visited. The results of the question on the frequency of visiting indicated that a substantial majority of family members saw their relatives in the nursing home quite often. We also asked the respondents about their relatives' level of mental awareness. The question was worded this way: "Many people in nursing homes have difficulty keeping track of things and knowing what is going on around them. How would you evaluate the mental awareness of your family member when you visit?" The four response categories ranged from "alert and aware all the time" to "rarely alert or aware."

In most cases it is impossible to determine with legal certainty exactly who, if anyone, is responsible when an item disappears from a patient's room in a nursing home. As stated earlier, items that disappear usually are explained away as having been simply lost, misplaced, or taken by other patients. To take account of these alternative explanations of theft, we developed a series of questions regarding the disappearance of items. We began by asking family members whether, in the past year, they had noticed any of their relatives' possessions missing. If they answered "yes," then we asked a series of questions about how many times they had noticed items missing and what they thought had happened. We asked if they suspected that the missing items were "lost or misplaced by the nursing home," and if so, how many times this had happened.

We asked the same questions in cases for which they suspected items were "inadvertently taken by other patients," "deliberately taken by other patients," "deliberately stolen by someone who was not an employee or patient," or "deliberately stolen by a nursing home employee." Family members could report multiple instances of items missing and could give different reasons for their disappearances. For example, a respondent could report that she had noticed two items missing in the past year, and she thought that one item had simply been lost while the other item was stolen by an employee. By giving respondents the opportunity to choose other nontheft scenarios, we hoped to arrive at a conservative estimate of the rate of victimization in nursing homes.

Glossary

abuse: The willful infliction of injury, unreasonable confinement, intimidation, or punishment with resulting physical harm, pain, or mental anguish. (Centers for Medicare and Medicaid Services)

active neglect: Intentionally not fulfilling caregiving obligations.

almshouses: In existence since up to the mid-1930s, they housed poor, aged, and infirm persons. (Also called poor farms, poor houses.)

Alzheimer's disease: A progressive brain disorder affecting thought, language, and memory. (*See also* DEMENTIA.)

American Association of Retired Persons (AARP): The nation's largest voluntary association for people age fifty and older. It serves their needs and interests through information and education, advocacy, and community services.

assisted living facility: A residential care home not licensed or certified as a nursing home that is usually licensed by the state and provides shelter and care to people with impairments or needs for routine nursing care.

autonomy: The control of decision making and over other activities of one's life and care. The autonomy of nursing home patients is sometimes highly restricted and comprised.

Boren Amendment: Enacted in 1980 and repealed in 1996, this law required states to reimburse nursing homes at a rate sufficient to meet quality standards.

bureaucracy: A hierarchical, formal, large-scale organization that operates under certain rules and procedures.

burnout: A syndrome characterized by emotional stress and exhaustion, resulting in a decline in the quality of patient care.

certified nursing aide (CNA): One who has successfully completed a training course of not less than seventy-five hours and has passed a practical examination.

chemical restraints: Drugs given to patients for behavioral and psychiatric problems.

decubitus ulcers: Skin lesions resulting from unrelieved pressure, which causes damage to the underlying tissue. Commonly called pressure sores or bedsores.

dementia: A general term for a decline in mental functioning which includes impairment of memory, orientation, and judgment. Alzheimer's is the most common disease associated with dementia.

depersonalization: The act of treating a patient as if he or she is a non-person without an identity.

depression: A frequent function disorder of old age that occurs with varying degrees of intensity and duration. Psychological characteristics of depression include discouragement, a sense of uselessness, and pessimism about the present and future.

deviant behavior: The violation of a significant social norm, especially one of the mores.

elder mistreatment: This term includes physical, psychological, material, and financial abuse as well as neglect. (*See also* ABUSE.)

ethnographic study: This type of research provides a rich description of how organizations work and how the research subjects view the world.

exploitation: Manipulating a patient's property for the benefit of others.

fair ratio: Based on the strain theory, this model proposes that employees in an organization expect to be fairly paid for the work that they do.

financial abuse: The theft or improper use of a patient's money by others.

general theory of crime: This theory posits that crime occurs when low self-control is combined with criminal opportunity.

gerichair: A type of restraint comprised of a chair with a tray attached that prevents the patient from being able to get up.

identity theft: The wrongful acquisition and use of one's personal data in a fraudulent manner for financial gain.

infantilization: The act of treating older people as children instead of as mature adults.

learned helplessness: A fatalistic passive attitude of accepting whatever comes along and a belief that all is hopeless.

licensed practical nurse (LPN): One who has graduated from an approved nursing program (usually one year long) that is licensed according to state requirements.

long-term care: Assistance given over a period of time to those who have difficulty in functioning because of a chronic disability.

material abuse: The theft or improper use of a patient's possessions.

Medicaid: A state-operated and state-administered program that is financed by the state and federal governments that provides medical benefits to low-income individuals. It pays about 68 percent of the nursing home expenses in the United States.

Medicare: A national health insurance program for people sixty-five and over and some disabled persons under age sixty-five. It has two parts: Part A is hospital insurance, which most persons do not have to pay for, and Part B is medical insurance, which most persons pay for monthly.

neglect: *See* ACTIVE NEGLECT; PASSIVE NEGLECT.

norms: Shared rules that prescribe the appropriate behavior in a given situation.

nursing aides (nurse's aides, nurse assistants): Persons who provide the bulk of care and assistance to nursing home patients and who are supervised by nurses.

nursing aides' registry: Each state keeps a record of all aides who have been cited for patient mistreatment.

nursing home: A facility with three or more beds that is licensed as a nursing home by the state and provides nursing care services.

nursing home reforms: These reforms are contained in the Omnibus Budget Reconciliation Act of 1987 (OBRA 1987). (*See also* OMNIBUS BUDGET RECONCILIATION ACT OF 1987 [OBRA '87].)

Older Americans Act: Passed in 1965, this act was created to provide an array of services and programs to foster the independence of older persons.

ombudsperson: Mandated by the Older Americans Act, this program requires each state to have a long-term care ombudsman to serve as an advocate for the need and interests of nursing home patients and to help defuse some of the problems related to their abuse and neglect.

Omnibus Budget Reconciliation Act of 1987 (OBRA '87): This legislation included a measurement of quality of care in nursing homes, developed new standards for residents' rights, and helped to reduce the use of physical and chemical restraints. It required each state to ensure quality services from nursing homes that are certified by Medicare and Medicaid.

passive neglect: Unintentionally not fulfilling caregiving obligations.

physical abuse: Acts that cause pain or injury.

physical restraints: Any device, material, or equipment attached to or near a patient's body that cannot be easily removed and that restricts freedom of motion or normal access to one's own body.

preemployment screening: A way of identifying unsuitable workers in order to protect vulnerable populations such as the elderly.

pressure sores: *See* DECUBITUS ULCERS.

psychoactive drugs: Mind-altering drugs that are used to control behavioral symptoms that affect thinking, feeling, and reacting.

psychological abuse: The causing of emotional pain or the threat of injury.

reactive abuser: One who commits an abusive act without planning or malicious intent.

routine activities theory: This theory maintains that three factors must converge for criminal activity to occur: suitable targets, absence of protection, and motivated offenders.

sadistic abuser: One who commits an abusive act with planning and malicious intent.

self-fulfilling prophecy: A prediction that starts a chain of events, which in turn makes the prediction come true.

self-report survey: A data-collection method relying on respondents to disclose their personal behaviors.

Senior Crimestoppers: A program that provides lockboxes for each patient in a participating nursing home. The boxes are mounted in the patients' rooms so that they can secure some of their possessions. The program also offers access to a tip hotline for reporting theft.

sexual abuse: Engaging in sexual contact with a person without his or her consent.

situational theory: As certain situational and/or structural factors increase for the abuser, the risk of abusive acts directed at a vulnerable patient who is seen as being related to the stress also increases.

total institution: Places of residence where a large number of like-situated individuals are cut off from the wider society for an appreciable length of time. (Goffman, 1961)

trust account: The personal allowance of a nursing home patient.

References

American Association of Retired Persons (1991). *Fact sheet on nursing homes.* Washington, DC: AARP.

American Association of Retired Persons (1998). *Nursing home life: A guide for residents and families.* Washington, DC: AARP.

American Association of Retired Persons (1999). *The states.* Washington, DC: AARP.

American Health Care Association (2001). *Facts and trends: The nursing facility sourcebook.* Washington, DC: Author.

Ansello, E.F. (1996). Causes and theories. In L.A. Baumhover and S.C. Beal (Eds.), *Abuse, neglect, and exploitation of older persons: Strategies for assessment and intervention* (pp. 9-29). Baltimore, MD: Health Professions Press.

Bonnie, R.J. and Wallace, R.B. (Eds.) (2003). *Elder mistreatment: Abuse, neglect, and exploitation in an aging America.* Washington, DC: National Academies Press.

Booth, B., Bruno, A., and Marin, R. (1996). Therapy with abused and neglected patients. In L. Baumhover and S.C. Beall (Eds.), *Abuse, neglect and exploitation of older person* (pp. 185-203). Baltimore, MD: Health Professions Press.

Bowers, B. and Becker, M. (1992). Nurse's aides in nursing homes: The relationship between organization and quality. *The Gerontologist, 32,* 360-366.

Brannon, D. (1992). Toward second-generation nursing home research. *The Gerontologist, 32,* 293-294.

Braun, K.L., Suzuki, K.M., Cusick, C.E., and Howard-Carhart, K. (1997). Developing and testing training materials on elder abuse and neglect for nurse aides. *Journal of Elder Abuse and Neglect, 9,* 1-15.

Burger, S.G., Fraser, V., Hunt, S., and Frank, B. (2000). *Nursing homes: Getting good care there.* Atascadero, CA: Impact Publishers, Inc.

Burns, F. (2000). Elderly patients victimized by identity theft. *APB News.*

The Center for Advocacy for the Rights and Interests of the Elderly (CARIE). (1999). Competence with compassion: An abuse prevention training program for long-term care staff. Philadelphia, PA: CARIE.

Centers for Medicare and Medicaid Services (2002). *Appropriateness of minimum staffing ratios in nursing homes.* Report to Congress. Baltimore, MD. Author.

Chan, S. (2002). Former D.C. nurse aide is charged in death. *Washington Post,* March 22.

Chappell, N. and Novak, M. (1992). The role of support in alleviating stress among nursing assistants. *The Gerontologist, 32,* 351-359.

Clarke, R. (1995). Situational crime prevention: Its theoretical basis and practical scope. In M. Tonry and N. Morris (Eds.), *Crime and justice: An annual review of research,* vol. 4 (pp. 91-150). Chicago: The University of Chicago Press.

Cohen, L.E. and Felson, M. (1979). Social change and crime rate trends. *American Sociological Review, 44,* 588-608.

Crime and Justice (2001). *The Washington Post,* April 4, p. B2.

Dey, A.N. (1997). *Characteristics of elderly nursing home residents: Data from the 1995 national nursing home survey. Advance data from vital and health statistics; no. 289.* Hyattsville, MD: National Center for Health Statistics.

Dunlop, D.D. (1979). *The growth of nursing home care.* Lexington, MA: D.C. Heath and Company.

Elrick, M. (2000). Thirteen charged in theft of seniors' names. *Detroit Free Press,* October 17.

Feldman, P. (1994). "Dead end" work or motivating job? Prospects for frontline paraprofessional workers in LTC. *Generations, 28,* 5-10.

Foner, N. (1994). *The caregiving dilemma: Work in an American nursing home.* Berkeley: University of California Press.

Foote, J. (1995). Final indignities: The care of elders with dementia. *Intelligence Journal,* May 19, p. C1.

Frontline Publishing Corp. (n.d.). *Nursing Assistant Monthly.* Somerville, MA: Frontline Publishing Corp.

Goergen, T. (2001). Stress, conflict, elder abuse and neglect in German nursing homes: A pilot study among professional caregivers. *Journal of Elder Abuse and Neglect, 13,* 1-26.

Goffman, E. (1961). *Asylums.* New York: Doubleday.

Goodridge, D., Johnston, P., and Thomson, M. (1996). Conflict and aggression as stressors in the work environment of nursing assistants: Implications for institutional elder abuse. *Journal of Elder Abuse and Neglect, 8,* 49-67.

Gottfredson, M.R. and Hirschi, J. (1990). *A general theory of crime.* Stanford: Stanford University Press.

Gubrium, J.F. (1975). *Living and dying at Murray Manor.* New York: St. Martin's Press.

Harris, D. (1988). *Dictionary of gerontology.* New York: Greenwood Press.

Harris, D. (1999). Elder abuse in nursing homes: The theft of patients' possessions. *Journal of Elder Abuse and Neglect, 10,* 141-151.

Harris, D. and Benson, M. (1997). Nursing home theft: The hidden problem. *Journal of Aging Studies, 12,* 57-67.

Harris D. and Benson, M. (1999). Theft in nursing homes: An overlooked form of elder abuse. *Journal of Elder Abuse and Neglect, 11,* 73-90.

Heine, C. (1986). Burnout among nursing home personnel. *Journal of Gerontological Nursing, 12,* 14-18.

Henderson, J.N. (1994). Bed, body, and soul: The job of the nursing home aide. *Generations, 18,* 20-27.

Hindelang, M., Hirschi, T., and Weis, J. (1981). *Measuring delinquency.* Beverly Hills, CA: Sage Publications.

Hodge, P. (1998). National law enforcement programs to prevent, detect, investigate, and prosecute elder abuse and neglect in health care facilities. *Journal of Elder Abuse and Neglect, 9,* 23-41.

Hollinger, R. and Clark, J. (1983). *Theft by employees.* Lexington, MA: Lexington Books.

Johnson, C. (1992). Coping with compassion fatigue. *Nursing, 22,*116-119.

Jones, A. (2000). The national nursing home survey: 1999 summary. National Center for Health Statistics 13(152).

Kamen, A. (2000). Victims of crime: Issues and patterns. In J. Shelley (Ed.), *Criminology: A contemporary handbook* (pp. 165-185). Belmont, CA: Wadsworth.

Kane, R.A., Kane, R.L., and Ladd, R.C. (1998). *The heart of long-term care.* New York: Oxford University Press.

Kayser-Jones, J. (1981). *Old, alone, and neglected.* Berkeley: University of California Press.

Kayser-Jones, J., Schell, E., Lyons, W., Kris, A.E., Chan, J., and Beard, R.L. (2003). Factors that influence end-of-life care in nursing homes: The physical environment, inadequate staffing, and lack of supervision. *The Gerontologist, 43,* 76-84.

Keller, B. (1996). A model abuse prevention training program for long-term care staff. In L.A. Baumhover and S.C. Beall (Eds.), *Abuse, neglect and exploitation of older persons* (pp. 221-239). Baltimore, MD: Health Professions Press.

Kimsey, L., Tarbox, A., and Bragg, D. (1981). Abuse of the elderly: The hidden agenda. *Journal of the American Geriatrics Society, 29,* 465-472.

Kosberg, I. and Nahmiash, D. (1996). Characteristics of victims and perpetrators. In L.A. Baumhover and S.C. Beal (Eds.), *Abuse, neglect, and exploitation of older people: Strategies for assessment and intervention* (pp. 31-49). Baltimore, MD: Health Professions Press.

Lab, S. and Allen, R. (1984). Self report and official measures: A further examination of the validity issue. *Journal of Criminal Justice, 12,* 445-455.

Lescoe-Long, M. (2000).Why they leave: A new approach to staff retention. *Nursing Homes,* October, 70-74.

Malone, J. (2000). Study overseers ignore nursing home complaints. *The Atlanta Constitution,* November 20, p. D1.

Meddaugh, D. (1993). Covert elder abuse in the nursing home. *Journal of Elder Abuse and Neglect, 5,* 21-37.

Menio, D. and Keller, B. (2000). CARIE: A multifaceted approach to abuse prevention in nursing homes. *Generations, 24,* 28-32.

Minority Staff of the House Committee on Government Reform (2001). *Abuse of residents is a major problem in U.S. nursing homes.* Washington, DC: U.S. House of Representatives.

Mitty, E. (2001). *The Encyclopedia of Aging,* Third edition. New York: Springer Publishing Co.

Munz, M. (2001a). Ex-official of nursing home admits theft, forgery she stole from resident after the woman died. *St. Louis Post-Dispatch,* May 2, p. B1.

Munz, M. (2001b). Former nursing home employee gets 15 years for abuse of patient. *St. Louis Post-Dispatch,* February 24, p. 8.

Munz, M. (2004). Ex-director of Claywest faces trial on failure to report abuse. Knowledge of threat is alleged in death of patient at home. Examiner's conclusion: Homicide. *St. Louis Post-Dispatch,* February 24.

National Citizens' Coalition for Nursing Home Reform. (2001a). Fact sheets: Residents' rights. Available at <nccnhr.newc.com>.

National Citizens' Coalition for Nursing Home Reform. (2001b). Newsletter, p. 1, December.

Nelson, K. (2001). Another option. *The Knoxville News-Sentinel,* October 8, pp. 1, 12.

Newbern, V. (1987). Caregiver perceptions of abuse in health care settings. *Holistic Nurse Practitioner, 1,* 64-74.

The NewsHour with Jim Lehrer/Kaiser Family Foundation/Harvard School of Public Health (2001). *National survey on nursing homes.* Available at <www.kff.org>.

Noelker, L. and Harel, Z. (2001). Humanizing long-term care: Forging a link between quality of care and quality of life. In S. Noelker and Z. Harel (Eds.), *Linking quality of long-term care and quality of life* (pp. 3-26). New York: Springer Publishing Co.

O'Brien, M.E. (1989). *Anatomy of a nursing home: A new view of resident life.* Owing Mills, MD: National Health Publishing.

Osgood, N., Brant, B., and Lipman, A. (1991). *Suicide among the elderly in long-term care facilities.* Westport, CT: Greenwood Press.

Pasupathi, M. and Lockenhoff, C. (2002). Ageist behavior. In T. Nelson (Ed.), *Ageism* (pp. 201-246). Cambridge, MA: MIT Press.

Payne, B.K. and Cikovic, R. (1995). An empirical examination of the characteristics, consequences, and causes of elder abuse in nursing homes. *Journal of Elder Abuse and Neglect, 7,* 61-74.

Pear, R. (2002). 9 to 10 nursing homes in U.S. lack adequate staff, a government study finds. *The New York Times,* February 18, A11.

Penner, L., Lydenia, K., and Mead, G. (1984) staff attitudes: Image or reality? *Journal of Gerontological Nursing, 10,* 110-117.

Pillemer, K. and Bachman-Prehn, R. (1991). Helping and hurting: Predictors of maltreatment of patients in nursing homes. *Research on Aging, 13,* 74-75.

Pillemer, K. and Hudson, B. (1993). A model abuse prevention program for nursing assistants. *The Gerontologist, 33,* 128-131.

Pillemer, K., Menio, D., and Hudson Keller, B. (2001). *Abuse-proofing your facility.* Somerville, MA: Frontline Publishing Corp.

Pillemer, K. and Moore, D. (1989). Abuse of patients in nursing homes: Findings from a survey of staff. *The Gerontologist, 29,* 314-320.

Podnieks, E. (1987). The victimization of older persons. *Canadian Journal of Psychiatric Nursing, 28,* 6-11.

Provider Magazine (1997). Washington, DC: American Health Care Association.

Ramsey-Klawsnik, H. (1995). Investigating suspected elder mistreatment. *Journal of Elder Abuse and Neglect, 7,* 41-67.

Ramsey-Klawsnik, H. (1996). Assessing physical and sexual abuse. In L.A. Baumhover and S.C. Beall (Eds.), *Abuse, neglect, and exploitation of older persons* (pp. 67-87). Baltimore, MD: Health Professions Press.

Ramsey-Klawsnik, H. (2000). Elder-abuse offenders: A typology. *Generations, 24,* 17-22.

Reinharz, S. (1986). Loving and hating one's elders: Twin themes in legend and literature. In K.A. Pillemer and R.S. Wolf (Eds.), *Elder abuse: Conflict in the family* (pp. 25-48). Dover, MA: Auburn House.

Rogers, P. (1996). Thieves prey on nursing home residents. *Miami Herald,* November 25, p. 1.

Rowden, T. (2000). Male nurse pleads no contest to charge that he had sex with patient. *St. Louis Post-Dispatch,* November 11, p. 3.

Sampson, R. (1987). Communities and crime. In M. Gottfredson and T. Hirschi (Eds.), *Positive criminology* (pp. 91-114). Newbury Park, CA: Sage.

Savishinsky, J.S. (1991). *The ends of time: Life and work in a nursing home.* New York: Bergin and Garvey.

Schlichter, J. (2000). Man pleads guilty to stealing from elderly victims. *Daily News,* January 7.

Seligman, M. (1975). *Helplessness.* San Francisco: W. H. Freeman.

Sengstock, M. and Steiner, S. (1996). Accessing nonphysical abuse. In L. Baumhover and S.C. Beall (Eds.), *Abuse, neglect and exploitation of older persons* (pp. 105-122). Baltimore, MD: Health Professions Press.

Shaw, M.M. (1998). Nursing home resident abuse by staff: Exploring the dynamics. *Journal of Elder Abuse and Neglect, 9,* 1-21.

Shield, R. (1988). *Uneasy endings: Daily life in an American nursing home.* Ithaca, NY: Cornell University Press.

Sieroshevski, W. (1896). Quoted in S. de Beavoir, *The coming of age* (New York: G.P. Putnam's Sons), 1972.

Sinclair, M. (1990). Demanding a right to security. *Washington Post,* December 18.

Soloman, K. (1983). Victimization by health professionals and the psychologic response of the elderly. In J. Kosberg (Ed.), *Abuse and maltreatment of the elderly* (pp. 150-171). Boston: John Wright.

Stannard, C. (1973). Old folks and dirty work: The social conditions for patient abuse in a nursing home. *Social Problems, 20,* 329-342.

Strahan, G. (1997). *An overview of nursing homes and their current residents: Data from the 1995 National Nursing Home Survey. Advance data from vital and health statistics; no. 290.* Hyattsville, MD: National Center for Health Statistics.

Teaster, P.B., Roberto, K.A., Duke, J.O., and Kim, M. (2000). Sexual abuse of older adults: Preliminary findings of cases in Virginia. *Journal of Elder Abuse and Neglect, 12,* 1-16.

Tellis-Nyak, V. and Tellis-Nyak, M. (1989). Quality of care and the burden of two cultures: When the world of the nurse's aide enters the world of the nursing home. *The Gerontologist, 29,* 307-313.

United States General Accounting Office (2002). *Nursing homes: More can be done to protect residents from abuse.* GAO-02-312. Washington, DC: Author.

U.S. Department of Justice (1998). *Guidelines for the screening of persons working with children, the elderly, and individuals with disabilities in need of support.* Washington, DC: Office of Juvenile Justice and Delinquency Prevention.

Vinton, L. and Mazza, N. (1994). Aggressive behavior directed at nursing home personnel by residents' family members. *The Gerontologist, 34,* 528-533.

Waxman, H., Carner, E., and Berkenstock, G. (1984). Job turnover and job satisfaction among nursing home aides. *The Gerontologist, 24,* 503-509.

Weber, M. (1922). *Economy and society.* Ephraim Fishoff et al. (transl.), 1968. New York: Bedminster Press.

Whitaker, C. Elderly victims. (1987). Bureau of Justice Statistics Special Report. Washington, DC: U.S. Government office.

Wilbur, K.W. and Reynolds, S.L. (1996). Introducing a framework for defining financial abuse of the elderly. *Journal of Elder Abuse and Neglect, 8,* 61-80.

Wilner, M. (1994). Working it out: Support groups for nursing assistants. *Generations, 28,* 39-40.

Woman pleads guilty. (2001) *The Troy Messenger,* January 7. Available at <http://www.troymessenger.com/articles/2001/01/07/export3596.txt>.

Wunderlich, G.S., Sloane, F.A., and Davis, C.K. (Eds.) (1996). *Nursing staff in hospitals and nursing homes: Is it adequate?* Washington, DC: National Academy Press.

Yamada, Y. (2002). Profile of home care aides, nursing home aides, and hospital aides: Historical changes and dat recommendations. *The Gerontologist, 42.*

Index

Page numbers followed by the letter "f" indicate figures; those followed by the letter "e" indicate exhibits; and those followed by the letter "t" indicate tables.